SpringerBriefs in Public Health

SpringerBriefs in Public Health present concise summaries of cutting-edge research and practical applications from across the entire field of public health, with contributions from medicine, bioethics, health economics, public policy, biostatistics, and sociology.

The focus of the series is to highlight current topics in public health of interest to a global audience, including health care policy; social determinants of health; health issues in developing countries; new research methods; chronic and infectious disease epidemics; and innovative health interventions.

Featuring compact volumes of 50 to 125 pages, the series covers a range of content from professional to academic. Possible volumes in the series may consist of timely reports of state-of-the art analytical techniques, reports from the field, snapshots of hot and/or emerging topics, elaborated theses, literature reviews, and in-depth case studies. Both solicited and unsolicited manuscripts are considered for publication in this series.

Briefs are published as part of Springer's eBook collection, with millions of users worldwide. In addition, Briefs are available for individual print and electronic purchase.

Briefs are characterized by fast, global electronic dissemination, standard publishing contracts, easy-to-use manuscript preparation and formatting guidelines, and expedited production schedules. We aim for publication 8–12 weeks after acceptance.

More information about this series at https://link.springer.com/bookseries/10138

Manako Yabe

Deaf Rhetoric

An Ecology of Health Communication

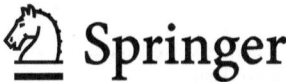 Springer

Manako Yabe
Faculty of Human Sciences
Division of Disability Sciences
University of Tsukuba
Tsukuba, Ibaraki, Japan

ISSN 2192-3698   ISSN 2192-3701   (electronic)
SpringerBriefs in Public Health
ISBN 978-3-030-96244-9   ISBN 978-3-030-96245-6   (eBook)
https://doi.org/10.1007/978-3-030-96245-6

This Springer imprint is published by the registered company Springer Nature Switzerland AG
The registered company address is: Gewerbestrasse 11, 6330 Cham, Switzerland

*This book is dedicated to those who have
contributed a piece of
the puzzle in my book journey.*

Preface

One day, I was playing on the grounds of my preschool. Suddenly, my father came and took me to the hospital. I did not know what had happened. In the scene before me lay my mother with a very pained and tear-stained face. Her mouth was covered with an oxygen mask. Her thin left wrist had an intravenous drip. She was in critical condition. My mother saw a bright light and was free from pain. She was ready for heaven. But at that moment, when her eyes caught my brother and me, who were 6 and 5 years old, she did not want to die and leave us. The light was gone, and the pain returned. She screamed and burst into tears.

Even at the age of five, I clearly remember the day when I encountered the lack of healthcare communication access in hospitals. The doctors and nurses discussed something with my father and grandmother in the room, but my brother and I could not understand what they were saying because we are deaf. Yet, I knew only one thing. Something was wrong. When I was seven, I finally understood what had happened in the hospital room. *My mother was so close to dying.*

Being Isolated in Healthcare Communication Access Settings

I was born deaf. My brother, also born deaf, is 1 year older. Our parents are hearing. At the time I was born in Japan in the 1980s, Japanese deaf education prohibited using Japanese Sign Language (JSL) as a method of instruction. Instead, it was popular to teach deaf children by using the "oral method," i.e., educating them through oral language. The use of JSL at deaf schools was slowly recognized and eventually accepted in the 1990s. Accordingly, my brother and I were initially educated through the "oral" approach.

Since my family wanted to seek better education for us, we moved to various locations across three countries, including: Japan (Tokyo), the UK (London), and the USA (Atlanta). In Japan, when I would go to the hospital, I always depended on my parents for translation from oral language into Japanese. When I was seven, we moved to Atlanta, and we lived there for 2 years. I attended a Japanese school, yet I still depended on my parents for translation from oral English language into

Japanese, while my parents spoke English with my audiologist. At that time, I was so fearful of English because I could not hear, speech-read, or completely understand spoken English. Consequently, I always relied on my parents when someone spoke to me in English.

When I was 14, we moved to London, and I lived there for 5 years. Again, I attended a Japanese school. Outside of school, I started learning British Sign Language (BSL) and eventually became comfortable learning written English. However, I was unable to speech-read and fully understand spoken English. Specifically, I could understand basic BSL, but I was not fluent in writing English. As a result, in healthcare settings, I depended on my parents' translation from oral English language into Japanese, while my parents attempted to understand my doctor's English, as a non-native language. At the time, I was ignorant to the fact that what I was experiencing was not full communication access that hearing people typically enjoyed. Luckily, my treatments were non-critical, and the lack of healthcare communication did not seriously impact my life.

Finally, I moved to the USA on my own and lived in Los Angeles and Chicago for more than a decade. My first exposure to a full English communication environment was in college. Eventually, I became fluent in English and American Sign Language (ASL). I used to go to my university clinic once or twice a year, as the clinic already had a sign language interpreter service. However, it was not until I was a PhD student that I began to visit the clinic more frequently.

I clearly remember the day when I was involved in a car accident with multiple vehicles, and I was injured. I had to communicate with the other drivers, a police officer, and the ambulance staff in full *written communication*. I also had to use my videophone to call my insurance company in *ASL* and call my doctor for an appointment via text message. Then, I had an epiphany: *Imagine if I were not fluent in English and ASL and were unable to fully write and sign in English. Imagine if I could not fully understand English and were unable to fully communicate with the drivers, the police officer, the ambulance staff, and the doctor, due to my limited literacy in English and ASL.*

The car accident gave me an awareness of the importance of healthcare communication and health literacy. Subsequently, I received unexpected injuries, came down with various illnesses, and was in and out of hospitals for 2 years. I also experienced a wide spectrum of communication differences during this period, including writing, the use of a sign language interpreter, a video remote interpreter, and direct communication for the different treatments that I received. All of these experiences led to my dissertation: *Healthcare Providers' and Deaf Patients' Perspectives on Video Remote Interpreting: A Mixed Methods Study* (2019).

During my Ph.D. dissertation research, a healthcare provider took me to a clinic room for an interview, which was the same room where I had received my first physical therapy after the car accident. This location represented the beginning of my dissertation journey. Two years later, as a Ph.D. student, I returned to the same clinic. My eyes were full of tears, and I could not stop crying. Eventually, this experience led to the creation of this book.

Purpose of the Book

The purpose of this book is to guide current and prospective healthcare profession-als, hospital administrators, and medical interpreters in the USA (and internation-ally) toward better ways of communicating with Deaf and hard of hearing (D/HH) patients and sign language interpreters in healthcare settings. It also provides an overview of the healthcare communication issues facing healthcare professionals and D/HH patients and the advantages and disadvantages of using in-person inter-preters versus video remote interpreting (VRI). With new developments in technol-ogy, hospital administrators have popularized the use of VRI and reduced the number of in-person interpreting services, which have negatively impacted the qual-ity of medical interpreting services. The pandemic has also intensified the move toward more VRI, particularly in the USA.

To identify appropriate interpreting services for specific treatments, I focus on healthcare professionals' and D/HH patients' interpreting preferences for critical and non-critical care in the USA and offer a new theoretical framework, i.e., the Ecology of Health Communication, to contextualize and analyze these prefer-ences. The ecological matrix and its five analytical dimensions (i.e., physical-material, psychological, social, spatial, and temporal) can help readers to understand how each dimension influences healthcare professionals' and D/HH patients' inter-preting preferences as well as the treatment outcomes. This book concludes by rec-ommending prioritizing the use of an appropriate interpreter for specific treatments and allocating funds for in-person interpreters for critical care treatments.

This book also addresses a unique topic raised by an international deaf researcher from Japan who uses English and ASL as non-native languages. Previous books and research articles have covered D/HH patients and D/HH researchers' perspectives on interpreting D/HH patients' needs and mental health issues as well as resources for communication needs. Yet, these studies were carried out by American-born researchers. In addition, there have been no discussions that directly address health-care professionals' perspectives on healthcare communication, their interpreting preferences, and their experiences working with D/HH patients versus limited English proficiency (LEP) patients. Therefore, this book encourages readers to learn from the different lenses through which D/HH patients and healthcare professionals view the issue, recognizing how the appropriate use of interpreting services can impact the quality of patient–provider communication, treatment outcomes, and patients' well-being.

Additional factors make this book especially timely and useful. In fact, there have been few Deaf Studies and Disability Studies curricula available at medical schools in the USA. My research concludes that more than 50% of healthcare pro-fessionals have no training experience for appropriately treating D/HH patients using VRI. Moreover, although VRI is relatively inexpensive, easy, and quick to access, it often has technological issues such as poor network access, a small screen, and limited flexibility. Some patients, like those with a visual impairment, cognitive disability, or limited literacy, have needs that are not well met with the use of

VRI. Yet, many hospitals have attempted to completely eliminate in-person interpreting in favor of VRI, and this action has negatively impacted patient–provider communication.

Finally, my research does not focus on collecting stories from VRI companies or medical interpreters in the USA. However, VRI companies must improve the quality of VRI services and the training of VRI interpreters in order for D/HH patients to understand healthcare providers' perspectives and find their advocacy in healthcare access.

Chapter Previews

This book consists of five chapters: Chapter 1 (Deaf People and Healthcare Communication) provides guidance for healthcare professionals who work with D/HH patients and clients in medical settings. It addresses the following areas: disability justice principles, the use of People-First Language; different perspectives on deafness; definitions of deaf, hard of hearing, and Deaf; and deafness myths. Common issues in healthcare communication with D/HH patients are also discussed, along with the intersectionality and culture of patient–provider communication. Additionally, communication strategies for D/HH patients are examined.

Chapter 2 (What is an Ecology of Health Communication?) introduces the new theoretical framework: the Ecology of Health Communication (EHC). The idea of EHC begins with Margaret Syverson's (1999) *The Wealth of Reality: An Ecology of Composition* and its ecological matrix, which consists of five analytical dimensions: physical-material, social, spatial, psychological, and temporal. Considering EHC enables readers to understand how the five dimensions influence patient–provider communication, treatment outcomes, and healthcare experiences.

Chapter 3 (Deaf and Hard of Hearing Patients' Perspectives) introduces the narratives of eight D/HH patients' experiences with VRI and in-person interpreters, along with their interpreting preferences for critical and non-critical care. My research found that the D/HH patients preferred in-person interpreters for both critical and non-critical care in order to achieve effective communication, translation accuracy, and a human trust relationship. Ultimately, the D/HH patients stated that VRI was inferior to an in-person interpreter in terms of the outcomes of patient–provider communication.

Chapter 4 (Healthcare Professionals' Perspectives) introduces the narratives of eight healthcare professionals, their experiences with VRI and in-person interpreting, their experiences with treating D/HH and LEP patients, their interpreting preferences for critical and non-critical care, and their suggestions for improving VRI services. The majority of the healthcare professionals did not have Deaf cultural knowledge, but they recognized the importance of patient–provider communication.

Chapter 5 (Conclusion and Implications) concludes that financial concerns and hospital systems play a key role in the choice of interpreting modality and the quality of medical interpreting services. My research also urges hospital administrators not to employ VRI on a widespread basis, but to continue allocating some funding for in-person interpreting during clinical care encounters. Moreover, training is recommended for healthcare professional students, healthcare professionals, VRI companies, VRI interpreters, and D/HH patients and their families to improve patient–provider communication and well-being in health care.

Tsukuba, Japan   Manako Yabe

Acknowledgments

My book journey has been like the seeds from a Japanese white dandelion that finally blooms on a concrete street. The idea for "Deaf Rhetoric: An Ecology of Health Communication" began from a tiny seed that was planted when Dr. Philip Hayek assisted me with writing my dissertation. He also recommended me Dr. Margaret Syverson's book *The Wealth of Reality: An Ecology of Composition*. Then, during the summer of 2019, I had an idea: We should contact Dr. Syverson about her book! Although I made this happen, I was still trying to determine how to plant this seed in my garden, which took longer than expected.

After 1 year had passed, I participated in the 2020 International Professional Communication Conference, where I met Dr. Aimee Roundtree. She encouraged me to start writing a book based on my Ph.D. dissertation. Finally, I started digging the soil for the seed. Then, after Dr. Susan Burch provided me with her wisdom about writing a book manuscript, I searched for the right publisher and found Ms. Janet Kim, Senior Editor of Springer Nature. I was ready to water the soil. When my book proposal was accepted by Springer, it was like a sprout had suddenly come out of the soil after a long winter. My sprout was so hungry and ready to grow, so I fed it by immediately writing my book manuscript with the support of my personal editors, anonymous peer reviewers, and colleagues from the 2021 Rhetoric Society of America, the 2021 Rhetoric of Health and Medicine, and the 2021 Special Interest Group on Design of Communication of the Association for Computing Machinery.

In addition, my sprout was surrounded in full sunshine with my personal supporters: Ms. Lissa Moreno, who has read many of my papers for more than a decade; Dr. Paul Maiden, who encouraged me to "Fight on!" with a Trojan spirit; the late Dr. Barbara Boyd, who cheers me on from heaven; and my family, who helped me keep my colorful garden alive.

Now, my dandelion seeds have become blossoms. They are not ordinary yellow dandelions, but special white dandelions, called *Japanese white dandelions*. These dandelions are native to southern Japan, and I was very lucky to find them. My garden has become full of white dandelions, much like a snow garden. My dandelions cannot wait to fly into the blue sky!

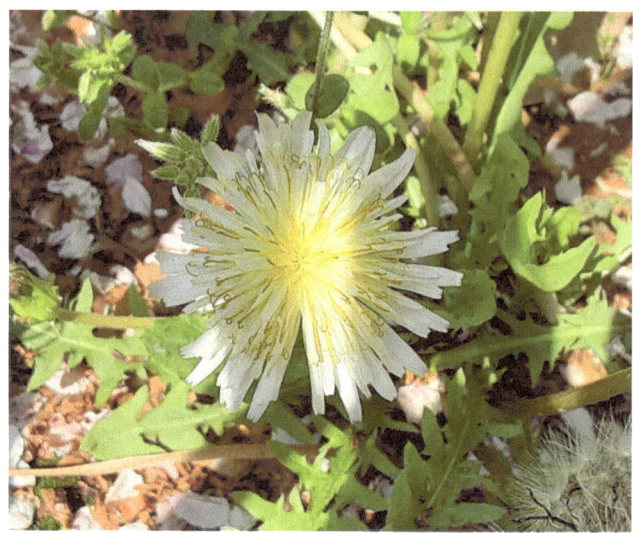

Photo credit: Manako Yabe, April 8, 2021, Kyoto, Japan

Contents

List of Figure

List of Tables

About the Author

Manako Yabe is the first Deaf faculty member in the Division of Disability Sciences at the University of Tsukuba, Japan. Dr. Yabe was born deaf in Japan and grew up in three countries: Japan, the UK, and the USA. She earned a Bachelor of Arts in Deaf Studies from California State University, Northridge, a Master's in Social Work from the University of Southern California, and a Doctor of Philosophy in Disability Studies from the University of Illinois, Chicago. Her areas of specialization include the following: Technical Communication, Deaf Studies, Disability Studies, Disability Rhetoric, Writing Center Studies, and Mixed Methods Research.

Abbreviations

ACA   Affordable Care Act
ADA   Americans with Disabilities Act
ASL   American Sign Language
BSL   British Sign Language
CDI   Certified deaf interpreter
D/HH   Deaf and hard of hearing
EHC   Ecology of Health Communication
JSL   Japanese Sign Language
LEP   Limited English proficiency
VRI   Video remote interpreting

Chapter 1

Deaf People and Healthcare Communication

As a foreign deaf patient, I have experienced the following at a healthcare appointment:
"Why do you need to use video remote interpreting? You can speak English."
"Because I am deaf, I need an interpreter to understand everything communicated during the MRI exam." The physician continued to resist writing and still spoke to me, but I decided to go on writing to the physician anyway. "Okay, please just tell me anything that I need to know before I go to sleep."
His tight face broke into a smile. He took my pen and wrote, "No, enjoy your dreams. I will let you know when the exam is done." Then, the physician continued writing me instructions about what would occur during my MRI.
My discomfort was gone, and I left the room with relief. That day was when I realized how important it was for a patient to educate a physician.

1.1 Introduction

Following this incident, I began looking for ways to educate physicians and medical students on the communication needs of deaf and hard of hearing (D/HH) patients. I felt that the issues in such situations come from a physician's "ignorance" of appropriate cultural competence with D/HH patients. Even though I have the privilege of holding a Ph.D., if I become a patient, then this privilege means nothing. In fact, the physicians and medical students I see have privilege over me. I cannot blame them for their "ignorance" because they have yet to receive appropriate training on how to treat D/HH patients. Thus, I often end up being silent and feeling disappointed.

Sadly, many medical schools do not offer Disability Studies or Deaf Studies curriculum. Meanwhile, many D/HH patients often feel frustration toward their physicians, in the same way that physicians may feel discomfort when seeing their D/HH patients (Borowsky et al., 2021). These issues have affected not only me, but also other limited English proficiency (LEP) patients in similar situations.

When I was a Ph.D. student at the University of Illinois, Chicago, I presented a Disability Studies workshop for the College of Dentistry. As a self-advocate, I joined the Illinois Leadership Education in Neurodevelopmental and Related Disabilities Program and discussed healthcare communication with D/HH patients.

M. Yabe, *Deaf Rhetoric*, SpringerBriefs in Public Health,
https://doi.org/10.1007/978-3-030-96245-6_1

I also developed a pilot Disability Studies curriculum for the College of Medicine, after which I received numerous comments about the importance of such training from medical students. Throughout my research, I was shocked to learn that most healthcare professionals did not receive any training in this area (Yabe, 2019).

Therefore, I decided to write this book to provide some resources on D/HH patients and healthcare communication. Although this book focuses on healthcare providers and D/HH patients in the USA, in particular, the information may also be helpful for those in other countries around the globe.

1.2 Ten Principles of Disability Justice

When I discuss healthcare communication with D/HH patients, I emphasize the importance of the Ten Principles of Disability Justice (Sins Invalid, 2017). This disability justice practice recognizes that individuals have different needs, backstories, and gifts, as well as complex and shifting identities. Given this recoginition, the common practice is to ask people how they would like to be identified and then follow their preferences. Additionally, these principles form an alliance that centers on disabled people as sources of valuable knowledge (Sins Invalid, 2017) (Table 1.1).

Table 1.1 Ten principles of disability justice

1. Intersectionality	"We are not only disabled, we are also coming from a specific experience of race, class, sexuality, age, religious background, geographical location, immigration status, and more"
2. Leadership of those Most impacted	"We keep ourselves grounded in real-world problems and find creative strategies for resistance"
3. Anti-capitalist politics	"The nature of our disabled bodyminds means that we resist conforming to 'normative' levels of productivly in a capitalist culture"
4. Cross-movement solidarity	"Through cross-movement solidarity, we create a united front"
5. Recognizing wholeness	"Disabled people are whole people"
6. Sustainability	"We value the teachings of our bodies and experiences, and use them as a critical guide and reference point to help us move away from urgency"
7. Cross-disability solidarity	"We value and honor the insights and participation of all of our community members, especially those who are most often left out of political conversations"
8. Interdependence	"We see the liberation of all living systems and the land as integral to the liberation of our own communities, as we all share one planet"
9. Collective access	"Access needs are not shameful—We function differently depending on the context and environment"
10. Collective liberation	"We move together as people with mixed abilities, multi-racial, multi-gendered, mixed class, across the sexual spectrum, with a vision that leaves no bodymind behind"

Sins Invalid (2017)

1.3 People-First Language

In my presentations, I also emphasize the importance of People-First Language and the etiquette of describing people with disabilities in appropriate language (Centers for Disease Control and Prevention [CDC], 2020a; Snow, 2016). As shown in Table 1.2, the term "handicapped persons" is no longer accepted, and "persons with disabilities" has become the appropriate language (CDC 2020a; Snow, 2016). However, disability activists strongly prefer Identity-First Language, since they want to be called "disabled people." While there have been different opinions across the broad community, the consensus is that they do not want to be called "the disabled" (American Psychological Association, 2021).

When I discuss D/HH patients, I use the phase "a deaf patient," not the words "mute, dumb, or hearing-impaired." Many deaf people prefer to be called "deaf people" rather than "a person who is deaf or hard of hearing" or "people with a hearing disability." Failing to use appropriate language can harm the human trust relationship between D/HH patients and healthcare professionals. Hence, it is essential to "recognize wholeness," i.e., the fifth disability justice principle, in order to see a deaf patient as a whole human.

A medical student once asked me the following questions: "Why it is okay to call a person visually impaired, while it is *not* okay to call another hearing-impaired?" and "Why it is *not* okay to say the person *overcomes* their disability?" The student brought up some great questions, and I explained that the disability community is a heterogeneous population. The Deaf community identify themselves as "deaf and hard of hearing" from a cultural perspective and "hearing-impaired" from a pathological perspective (National Center on Disability and Journalism, 2018). Taking a similar approach, the healthcare provider community uses inclusive language based on race and ethnicity, immigrant status, gender and sexual orientation, and ability in patient care and patient–provider communication (Oregon Health & Science University, 2021).

Table 1.2 People-first language

Use	Do not use
• Person with a disability, disabled person	• The disabled, handicapped
• Person without a disability, non-disabled person	• Normal person, healthy person
• Deaf, hard of hearing person	• Mute, dumb, hearing-impaired
• Person who is blind/visually impaired	• The blind
• Person with intellectual, cognitive, developmental disability	• Mentally retarded, moronic, slow
• Accessible parking or bathroom	• Handicapped parking or bathroom
• Person who is successful, productive	• Has overcome his/her disability, is courageous

American Psychological Association (2021) and Centers for Disease Control and Prevention (2020a)

1.4   Two Theoretical Lenses on Deafness

There are many different approaches to understanding disability and deafness, some of which significantly differ from the biomedical framework that dominates society in the USA in general, and the medicine and healthcare service field in particular. This book focuses on two frameworks: a Western biomedical model and a social-cultural model. In this section, I discuss two theoretical lenses on deafness: Deaf Studies and Disability Studies.

1.4.1   Deaf Studies

In general, the healthcare provider community and the Deaf community recognize deafness differently. The former is a dominantly hearing community, and its members may have no idea that they are "hearing people" or belong to "hearing society." In contrast, Deaf Studies focuses on the lives of Deaf people, including their culture, language, history, and human rights, rather than an auditory one (Marschark & Humphries, 2010). Additionally, Deaf Studies scholars spotlight two distinctly different ways that deafness and deaf people have been understood.

The healthcare provider community also focuses on the pathological perspective, i.e., the degree of hearing loss and how to correct it through cochlear implants and hearing aids or by learning speech and lip-reading. This perspective emphasizes making deaf persons become "hearing" as soon as possible because hearing is considered "normal" (McLeod & Bently, 1996).

In contrast, the cultural perspective focuses on deafness as a unique difference and does not see deafness as being "hearing-impaired" or a "deficit." Members of the Deaf community identify themselves as "deaf and hard of hearing people" from a cultural perspective and as a linguistic minority group (Padden & Humphries, 1988). Moreover, the Deaf community includes a wide variety of individuals who have varying degrees of hearing loss, use multiple languages, and belong to different physical cultures (Meador & Zazove, 2005).

Meanwhile, distinct definitions of Deaf, deaf, hard of hearing, and hearing exist within the Deaf community. Individuals who are considered "Deaf" are referred to as members of the Deaf community and use American Sign Language (ASL) as a primary language. "Deaf" individuals regard successful Deaf adults as role models, and the term empowers Deaf people as equal to hearing people (Padden & Humphries, 1988; National Association of the Deaf [NAD], 2021).

While "deaf" often refers to the audiological condition of not hearing and suggests seeking a "cure" for deafness, "hard of hearing" refers to a person with mild to moderate hearing loss. The hard of hearing person might or might not have any cultural affiliation with the Deaf community. Additionally, a "hearing" person might or might not be familiar with Deaf culture and ASL (Padden & Humphries, 1988; NAD, 2021). Nowadays, the field of Deaf Studies has been shifting its use of D/deaf. For example, some scholars are no longer use the uppercase D to designate the community's cultural identity and way of being, while other scholars include the word "culture" when relevant (Kusters et al., 2017).

The Deaf community has also discussed the understanding of the term "audism." In contrast, the "hearing society" focuses on the dependence on oral language and the belief in its superiority over signed languages. This is based on the assumption that being hearing is preferable to being deaf, and that deaf people want to or should be more like hearing people, indicating that deaf people have a defect, i.e., the inability to hear (Bauman, 2013; Gertz, 2007).

1.4.2   Disability Studies

Disability Studies use multiple theories to define disability and understand the disability experience from various interdisciplinary viewpoints (Rembis, 2010). For example, Kafer's (2013) political/relational theory of disability holds more space for disabled people who want and need medical access and treatment. However, it is still anchored to the belief that disability is not merely an objective deficit that needs a cure. Meanwhile, grassroots community members and Disability Studies scholars have introduced the social-cultural model and identified the medical model. However, they do not endorse the latter.

Traditionally, the medical model focuses on the individual with a disability (as a problem) and attempts to fix the impairment so that the person can become an able-bodied person and assimilate into the dominant society (Oliver, 1996). This model is similar in concept to the pathological perspective in Deaf Studies. The medical model also considers disability a tragedy for the individual and a burden for the family and society. Additionally, it focuses on the lack of physical, sensory, or mental functioning and views disability as an impairment, a form of victimization, or a problem (Democracy Disability and Society Group, 2003a).

In contrast, the social model focuses on society as a problem because it fails to design an accessible environment for people with disabilities. This model views environmental barriers as excluding persons with disabilities from full participation in society (Oliver, 1996). In this regard, it does not blame the individuals for the problem but identifies solutions to problems and removes barriers for people with disabilities, as an equal opportunity model. Moreover, it acknowledges the right of people with disabilities to full participation as citizens (Democracy Disability and Society Group, 2003b). Thus, it is not appropriate to say, "the person with a disability *overcomes* his/her disability." For instance, when a train station may make an emergency radio announcement, but a deaf person may be unable to access the information. In the social model, the train station is the party in which the problem is located because it failed to accommodate the deaf person with captioned emergency announcements. In the case of a medical setting, a hospital administrator may refuse to provide an in-person interpreter and insist on a video remote interpreter (VRI) for a D/HH patient. In this case, this action fails to respect the D/HH patient's interpreting preferences.

1.4.3   Understanding Legal Obligations Through Deaf Studies and Disability Studies Lenses

The Americans with Disabilities Act (ADA) ensures that people with disabilities receive accommodations in health care. However, this definition of disability is still rooted in the pathological perspective that deafness is a physical impairment (Donoghue, 2003; US Department of Justice, 2020). From this perspective, D/HH patients should request an interpreter to communicate with their healthcare professionals because they are unable to physically hear oral spoken language, and the healthcare professionals should provide interpreting services as a legal obligation under the ADA.

From the Deaf Studies' cultural perspective, healthcare professionals who are not fluent in ASL need an interpreter to communicate with D/HH patients. Since the purpose of using interpreting services is to build a bridge between D/HH patients and healthcare professionals and to overcome communication barriers, this viewpoint recognizes the barriers inherent for both parties. Hence, it is essential to advocate for language fluidity and rhetorical practices as "moments" of specific decision-making (Gonzales & Bloom-Pojar, 2018).

One Deaf Studies approach to interpreting recognizes the communication barriers that exist with D/HH patients and non-signing healthcare professionals. Yet, hospital administrators may decide to reduce the number of staff interpreters and make broad use of VRI interpreters out of financial considerations, rather than D/HH patients' communication preferences. As a result, D/HH patients may be unable to access staff interpreters and end up using VRI interpreters. This is an example of how "ableism" and "audism" shape hospital administration systems.

1.4.4   Myths of Deafness

When healthcare professionals and D/HH patients encounter cultural conflicts and miscommunication, it is not only due to a lack of Deaf cultural knowledge, but also belief in the myths of deafness. The following common myths are excerpted from the post "Myths about Deaf People" on the blog "If My Hands Could Speak…" (Anonymous, 2012):

All deaf people can read lips. Many hearing people have often asked me, "Can you lip-read?" Many deaf people cannot lip-read or cannot lip-read effectively enough to understand a conversation. In fact, it is estimated that lip-readers understand only approximately 30% of a conversation, with a lower rate in group conversations (Truman, 2020).

All people who are deaf will pass deafness on to their children. Historically, many deaf adults were banned from marrying other deaf people or endured forced sterilization without their consent (Womble & Jones, 2005). However, only 10% of deaf parents have deaf children, while 90% of deaf parents have hearing children (Mitchell & Karchmer, 2004).

Sign language is bad for deaf people. For a long time, deaf children were banned from using sign languages at deaf schools, both nationally and internationally (Bayton, 1996; Burch, 2002). However, sign languages have the same linguistic properties as spoken languages and a grammatical structure that differs from English (National Institute on Deafness and Other Communication Disorders [NIDCD], 2019a). Ironically, doctors have increasingly encouraged hearing babies to learn sign languages but typically discourage parents of deaf babies to learn sign language to communicate with their infants.

Sign language is universal. There is no universal sign language (NIDCD, 2019a). For instance, when I lived in Japan, I learned Japanese Sign Language; when I lived in the UK, I learned British Sign Language; and when I lived in the USA, I learned ASL. Each of these sign languages includes different finger spellings, signs, and grammatical structures.

People who are deaf cannot use the telephone. Due to new developments in technology, D/HH people have more opportunities to use assistive devices and programs such as text messaging, video relay services, and captioning services. These are often available via a remote interpreter (NIDCD, 2019b).

Hearing aids restore hearing. Assistive technology devices such as hearing aids and cochlear implants may enhance or enable an individual's hearing, but they may not make their hearing as functional as "normal" hearing (NIDCD, 2017).

People who are deaf are less intelligent. The inability to hear is unrelated to intelligence. In fact, 90% of deaf children are born to hearing parents, and the majority of hearing parents do not sign. Meanwhile, a lack of communication access and literacy development can impact deaf children's linguistic growth, and as a result, they experience "linguistic deprivation" (Harmer, 1999; Glickman & Hall, 2019; Mitchell & Karchmer, 2004).

1.5 Healthcare Communication Barriers with Deaf and Hard of Hearing Patients

In the USA, approximately 37.5 million adults report some degree of hearing loss (NIDCD, 2020). Hearing loss affects people of all ages and ranges from mild to profound. The causes of hearing loss vary, including temporary or permanent loss (NIDCD, 2020). Meanwhile, people with hearing loss have legal protections and rights to ensure communication access through Section 504 of the Rehabilitation Act of 1973 and the ADA of 1990 (US Department of Justice, 2020). The Department of Health and Human Services has also proposed a rule for the implementation of Section 1557 of the Affordable Care Act (ACA), which prohibits discrimination in health care (Cornachione et al., 2016).

Despite these legal protections, D/HH patients still encounter communication barriers for different reasons, including healthcare professionals' lack of cultural awareness and knowledge of legal obligations to D/HH patients, the unavailability of sign language interpreters, and D/HH patients' limited health literacy skills

(Desrosiers, 2017; Harmer, 1999; Meador & Zazove, 2005). Frequently, healthcare professionals have asked D/HH patients to bring their friends or family members (including their parents or children) to a medical appointment in order to help interpret the information (Harmer, 1999).

As stated earlier, 90% of D/HH patients' family members are hearing and are not fluent in sign language, resulting in D/HH patients having limited communication access at home (Mitchell & Karchmer, 2004). When deaf children with limited communication access at home visit their doctors with their parents, the parents and doctors have conversations that leave out the deaf children, thus excluding them from access to important information. As a result, deaf children never learn how to be involved as active patients, which can lead to their becoming passive patients in adulthood (Harmer, 1999). Related research has also found that D/HH patients have different communication modalities, and their sign languages have grammatical systems that differ from spoken languages (Iezzoni et al., 2004; Hoang et al., 2011).

Healthcare professionals might assume that it is sufficient to communicate with D/HH patients through speech reading or written communication. However, D/HH patients are not often fluent in speech reading or have a limited understanding of health literacy (Czerniejewski, 2012). In this regard, ignorance and misassumptions can cause communication barriers for D/HH patients, which may negatively affect their treatment outcomes and healthcare experiences.

Such communication and linguistic barriers can also reduce the quality of care and increase the risk of preventable adverse events such as unintended injuries or complications in the delivery of clinical care (Bartlett et al., 2008; Kuenburg et al., 2016). Meanwhile, some D/HH patients who are native signers struggle to understand spoken English due to their limited English literacy skills. Specifically, their use of communication and linguistic barriers do not allow them to gain knowledge about topics such as sexual health, cancer, preventive health care, and cardiovascular disease (McKee et al., 2011).

1.5.1 Healthcare Communication Barriers Associated with Cultural Conflict

Healthcare communication barriers are often associated with conflict between hearing and Deaf cultures in the intersectionality surrounding D/HH patients. In general, culture influences what people believe in relation to rituals, habits, laws, body image, sexuality, etc. These beliefs and attitudes have often been intricately linked to discrimination in the Deaf community (Lane, 1999). Additionally, the dominant hearing society may believe that Deaf people are abnormal and exclude them (Charlton, 1998; Lane, 1999). In this regard, healthcare professionals are referred to as members of a dominant hearing culture, while D/HH patients are referred to as members of a minority Deaf culture. According to previous research, members of the dominant and minority cultures might hold prejudiced attitudes toward the other (Harmer, 1999). Healthcare professionals may also make the misassumption that their deafness results in low intelligence or that D/HH patients are less intelligent than hearing patients (Iezzoni et al., 2004).

Due to cultural and linguistic differences, healthcare professionals might become concerned about the cost of providing interpreting services (Masland et al., 2010), or they might feel uncomfortable when working with D/HH patients (Hoang et al., 2011). Even when interpreters are available, some healthcare professionals might feel uncomfortable working directly with D/HH patients and only maintain eye contact with the interpreters, rather than their D/HH patients (Iezzoni et al., 2004). As a result, the D/HH patients can feel as if they are not treated with dignity and respect. Consequently, they might avoid visiting a doctor's office altogether (Iezzoni et al., 2004; Steinberg et al., 2002).

1.5.2   Healthcare Communication Barriers Associated with Intersectionality

Not only cultural conflicts, but also the intersectionality surrounding D/HH patients have been strongly associated with healthcare communication barriers. Intersectionality is defined as the intertwined nature of gender, race, class, ability, sexuality, and other social categories. Intersectionality has also been interwoven with the axes of oppression and discrimination (Wilkinson, 2003). Meanwhile, the interlocking systems of racism and ableism can create inequality based on culturally specific judgments of race and disability. Individuals may also experience discrimination from both axes of discrimination, due to racism and ableism (Wilkinson, 2003). In other words, D/HH patients encounter communication barriers not only because of ableist attitudes toward deafness, but also due to additional factors such as linguism, racism, sexism, transphobia, audism, and ableism (DeVault et al., 2011; Harmer, 1999).

LEP is a common factor associated with related communication barriers. Deaf patients who are ASL users tend to have LEP skills because they were either born deaf or lost their hearing during early childhood and then learned ASL with English as a second language. Other deaf patients use English as a primary language, but their English is not standard English (Barnett et al., 2011; Meador & Zazove, 2005). Additionally, D/HH patients with LEP often grow up in hearing families with members who are not fluent in sign language. As a result, such patients experience limited access to information regarding their health care and legal rights (Harmer, 1999; Steinberg et al., 2002). Healthcare professionals may be unaware that D/HH patients with LEP have limited communication access at home. Accordingly, they make the misassumption that D/HH patients are not intelligent because of their incorrect English (Iezzoni et al., 2004).

Race and ethnicity are also factors related to healthcare communication barriers. In fact, Deaf minority patients are more likely to experience limited healthcare access in comparison to Deaf White patients (Harmer, 1999). Similarly, Deaf women from minoritized racial and ethnic groups have the greatest difficulty accessing healthcare services, compared to Deaf White women (Harmer, 1999). These Deaf racially and ethnically minoritized patients have to negotiate three or more languages and cultures: the culture and language in their home; the culture and language of the Deaf community; and the culture and language of the dominant hearing community (Harmer, 1999).

Gender and socioeconomic status also play an important role in creating healthcare communication barriers. Compared to hearing women, Deaf women tend to have lower literacy rates, lower income, and higher unemployment rates. Since they may have limited family conversations and access to healthcare information, Deaf women are often unable to obtain basic preventive health care such as cancer screenings, mammograms, pap smears, or hormone replacement therapy (Steinberg et al., 2002).

Finally, embodied disability is the most common factor contributing to communication barriers. D/HH patients live in a paradoxical world in which they encounter obstacles to communication due to deafness or multiple disabilities. Often, they feel uncomfortable when healthcare professionals ask about the cause of their deafness even though it is not related to their actual health problems. As a result, D/HH patients and their families may feel ashamed and frustrated about their hearing loss (Iezzoni et al., 2004).

1.6 Advantages and Disadvantages Related to Interpreting Use

Since ASL is a different language than spoken English and most D/HH patients cannot effectively read lips, interpreters or captioning services are necessary to bridge the patient–provider communication gap. Therefore, Section 504 of the Rehabilitation Act of 1973, the ADA, and the ACA stipulate that healthcare providers must provide accommodations for D/HH patients (Cornachione et al., 2016; US Department of Justice, 2020). Furthermore, these legal obligations emphasize respecting D/HH patients' preferences regarding interpreting modality, not healthcare professionals' preferred choices.

Technological developments have also increased the popularity of VRI and led to a reduction in the number of in-person interpreters at hospitals (Desrosiers, 2017; Masland et al., 2010). However, it is imperative that healthcare professionals understand the advantages and disadvantages of VRI versus in-person interpreting for different clinical situations. They must also respect D/HH patients' interpreting preferences and provide equal access for their treatment.

1.6.1   Video Remote Interpreting

VRI is offered via a laptop or tablet that allows healthcare professionals and D/HH patients to communicate through a remote interpreter. A human interpreter appears live on the screen and interprets, instead of a computer interpreting by voice recognition (Alley, 2012). VRI has advantages over in-person interpreters, including 24-7 availability, cost-effectiveness, and usefulness for last-minute appointments (Masland et al., 2010). Nevertheless, it includes some disadvantages such as poor connectivity and visual and mobility limitations for placing the device in an effective position. In addition, VRI is not accessible for unique populations such as D/HH patients with cognitive disabilities, linguistic limitations, or mental disabilities, or those who are visually impaired (Rosenblum, 2015).

1.6.2   In-Person Interpreting

In-person interpreting has advantages over VRI in that it provides more accurate and effective translation (NAD, 2018). It also provides sufficient communication access for not only patients' needs but also healthcare professionals' needs (Bagchi et al., 2010). However, in-person interpreting services are comparatively more expensive and require advance notice to request/cancel an appointment (Masland et al., 2010). Additionally, budgetary and other concerns may limit the availability of in-person interpreters. Another obstacle related to both modalities is that healthcare professionals tend to have limited training on how to treat D/HH patients and the appropriate use of VRI or in-person interpreting (Yabe, 2019).

1.6.3   Lack of Training Availability

In the USA, there are limited Deaf Studies and Disability Studies curriculums at medical schools. One study found that more than 50% of healthcare professionals have no training in treating D/HH patients or using VRI (Yabe, 2019). Only a few healthcare providers, like speech-language pathologists who often work with D/HH patients, have received training with D/HH patients (Yabe, 2019). It appears that healthcare professionals only learn how to use VRI or to treat D/HH patients through their own treatment experiences, but not through training or academic studies at medical schools. Accordingly, like babies who learn how to walk by themselves without formal training, healthcare professionals have learned how to use VRI interpreters and how to treat D/HH patients in an unsystematic manner. While this method might be a good approach to learning, it can also produce negative effects in terms of patient–provider communication. Therefore, medical schools should require the learning of both practice and theory for treating D/HH patients, which can lead to better patient–provider communication and ultimately improve the quality of care.

1.7   Conclusion

This chapter emphasizes the importance of cultural competence training for medical students and healthcare professionals, an understanding of the different characteristics and communication needs of D/HH patients, and the ability to identify appropriate interpreting services for specific treatments. Many factors also shape communication access, including systems of power and privilege. Thus, recognizing that D/HH patients have many identities in addition to being deaf and addressing the full person in healthcare settings is an important part of effective care.

Appendix: Communication Strategies for Working with Deaf and Hard of Hearing Patients

It is essential to understand the advantages and disadvantages of interpreting services, deaf and hard of hearing (D/HH) patients' communication needs, and the legal obligation to provide communication accommodation. It is also critical to recognize the various aspects of the hearing culture and the Deaf culture, and to be aware of not only communication and language barriers, but also their intersectionality with language, race and ethnicity, gender, socioeconomic status, and disability.

Moreover, it is important to consider various communication strategies with these patients such as providing appropriate interpreting services, ensuring a clear visual field, refraining from sitting in front of a bright window, talking to the patient without overenunciating, and speaking directly to the patient rather than directing communication to the interpreter (Meador & Zazove, 2005).

The following tips are summarized from the training guide *Access to Medical Care* (Saxton et al., 2011).

Treating Deaf and Hard of Hearing Patients

When you treat patients who have identified themselves as "deaf" or "hard of hearing" and use English as a primary language, there are several things to consider:

First, please ask the patient how to best communicate with him/her and prepare to provide written educational materials while minimizing background noise and glare.

Second, please do not talk to the patient from a distance (or from another room), shout or exaggerate mouth movements, or talk rapidly. Simply look at the patient while speaking clearly in a normal tone of voice and make sure that he/she can see your mouth.

Third, since lip movement is only 30–40% visible, it is very difficult for a patient to speech-read medical terminology that is unfamiliar to them. Please draw on their capability to see the information such as by drawing pictures of symptoms, writing out medical terminology, using an interpreter for a group conversation, and removing your mask to allow the patient to see your facial expressions.

Treating Cultural Deaf Patients

When you treat patients who have identified themselves as culturally "Deaf" and use American Sign Language (ASL) or other sign languages as a primary language, there are several things to consider:

First, please ask the patient how best to communicate. The patient may request an interpreter who is an ASL interpreter, a Pidgin Sign English (PSE) interpreter, or a certified deaf interpreter (CDI). Each deaf individual has different communication preferences. PSE is a mixture of ASL and English, which differs from ASL as a distinct language (CDC, 2020b), while a CDI provides interpreting services to Deaf individuals who use other sign languages or have linguistic limitations that prevent them from understanding an ASL interpreter (National Consortium of Interpreter Education Center, 2014).

Second, hospitals are responsible for providing interpreting services. You should not charge the patient nor ask him/her to bring family members or friends for translation.

Third, avoid calling the patient "hearing-impaired." Please speak directly to the patient and do not say things to the interpreter like "Tell them…" Eye contact is essential for language access, and it respects Deaf cultural manners.

Finally, if the patient does not understand your instructions or questions, then repeat or use other words or find another approach to providing the information. Please take the necessary time to meet the patient's healthcare needs.

References

Alley, E. (2012). Exploring remote interpreting. *International Journal of Interpreter Education, 4*(1), 111–119. http://www.cit-asl.org/new/exploring-remote-interpreting/

American Psychological Association. (2021). *Disability*. https://apastyle.apa.org/style-grammar-guidelines/bias-free-language/disability

Anonymous. (2012). *Myths about deaf people*. https://ifmyhandscouldspeak.wordpress.com/common-myths-about-deaf-people-and-the-truth/

Bagchi, A. D., Dale, S., Verbitsky-Savitz, N., & Andrecheck, S. (2010). *Using professionally trained interpreters to increase patient/provider satisfaction: Does it work?* (Issue Brief No. 6). Mathematica Policy Research, Inc. https://www.issuelab.org/resources/11530/11530.pdf

Barnett, S., McKee, M., Smith, S. R., & Pearson, T. A. (2011). Deaf sign language users, health inequities, and public health: Opportunity for social justice. *Preventing Chronic Disease, 8*(2), A45. https://www.cdc.gov/pcd/issues/2011/mar/10_0065.htm

Bartlett, G., Blais, R., Tamblyn, R. J., Clermont, R., & MacGibbon, B. (2008). Impact of patient communication problems on the risk of preventable adverse events in acute care settings. *Canadian Medical Association, 178*(12), 1555–1562. https://doi.org/10.1503/cmaj.070690

Bauman, H. D. (2013). *Audism.* Encyclopedia Britannica. https://www.britannica.com/topic/audism

Bayton, D. C. (1996). *Forbidden signs.* University of Chicago Press.

Borowsky, H., Morinis, L., & Garg, M. (2021). Disability and ableism in medicine: A curriculum for medical students. *MedEdPORTAL: The Journal of Teaching and Learning Resources, 17*, 11073. https://doi.org/10.15766/mep_2374-8265.11073

Burch, S. (2002). *Signs of resistance.* New York University Press.

Centers for Disease Control and Prevention. (2020a). *Communicating with and about people with disabilities..* https://www.cdc.gov/ncbddd/disabilityandhealth/materials/factsheets/fs-communicating-with-people.html.

Centers for Disease Control and Prevention. (2020b). *Conceptually accurate signed English (CASE).* https://www.cdc.gov/ncbddd/hearingloss/parentsguide/building/case.html

Charlton, J. (1998). *Nothing about us without us: Disability oppression and empowerment.* University of California Press.

Cornachione, E., Musumeci, M., & Artiga, S. (2016). *Summary of HHS's final rule on nondiscrimination in health programs and activities* (Issue Brief). The Kaiser Commission on Medicaid and the Uninsured. https://files.kff.org/attachment/issue-brief-Summary-of-HHSs-Final-Rule-on-Nondiscrimination-in-Health-Programs-and-Activities

Czerniejewski, E. M. (2012). *A system to enhance patient–provider communication in hospitalized patients who use American sign language* [Master's thesis, University of Iowa]. Iowa Research Online. https://ir.uiowa.edu/cgi/viewcontent.cgi?referer=&httpsredir=1&article=3220&context=etd

Democracy Disability and Society Group. (2003a). *Medical model of disability.* http://ddsg.org.uk/taxi/medical-model.html

Democracy Disability and Society Group. (2003b). *Social model of disability.* http://ddsg.org.uk/taxi/social-model.html

Desrosiers, P. (2017). *Signed language interpreting in healthcare settings: Who is qualified?* Honors senior thesis, Western Oregon University. Digital Commons@WOU. https://digitalcommons.wou.edu/cgi/viewcontent.cgi?article=1123&context=honors_theses

DeVault, M., Garden, R., & Schwartz, M. A. (2011). Mediated communication in context: Narrative approaches to understanding encounters between health care providers and deaf people. *Disability Studies Quarterly, 31*(4) http://dsq-sds.org/article/view/1715/1763

Donoghue, C. (2003). Challenging the authority of the medical definition of disability: An analysis of the resistance to the social constructionist paradigm. *Disability and Society, 18*(2), 199–208. https://doi.org/10.1080/0968759032000052833

Gertz, G. (2007). Dysconscious audism: A theoretical proposition. In H. D. Bauman (Ed.), *Open your eyes: Deaf studies talking* (pp. 219–234). University of Minnesota Press.

Glickman, N. S., & Hall, W. C. (Eds.). (2019). *Language deprivation and deaf mental health.* Routledge.

Gonzales, L., & Bloom-Pojar, R. (2018). A dialogue with medical interpreters about rhetoric, culture, and language. *Rhetoric of Health and Medicine, 1*(1–2), 193–212. https://doi.org/10.5744/rhm.2018.1002

Harmer, L. M. (1999). Health care delivery and deaf people: Practice, problems, and recommendations for change. *Journal of Deaf Studies and Deaf Education, 4*(2), 73–110. https://doi.org/10.1093/deafed/4.2.73

Hoang, L., LaHousse, S. F., Nakaji, M. C., & Sadler, G. R. (2011). Assessing deaf cultural competency of physicians and medical students. *Journal of Cancer Education, 26*(1), 175–182. https://doi.org/10.1007/s13187-010-0144-4

Iezzoni, L. I., O'Day, B. L., Killeen, M., & Harker, H. (2004). Communicating about health care: Observations from persons who are deaf or hard of hearing. *Annals of Internal Medicine, 140*(5), 356–362. https://doi.org/10.7326/0003-4819-140-5-200403020-00011

Kafer, A. (2013). *Feminist queer crip*. Indiana University Press.

Kuenburg, A., Fellinger, P., & Fellinger, J. (2016). Health care access among deaf people. *Journal of Deaf Studies and Deaf Education, 21*(1), 1–10. https://doi.org/10.1093/deafed/env042

Kusters, A. M. J., De Meulder, M., & O'Brien, D. (Eds.). (2017). *Innovations in deaf studies: The role of deaf scholars*. Oxford University Press.

Lane, H. (1999). *The mask of benevolence: Disabling the deaf community*. Dawn Sign Press.

Marschark, M., & Humphries, T. (2010). Deaf studies by any other name? *Journal of Deaf Studies and Deaf Education, 15*(1), 1–2. https://doi.org/10.1093/deafed/enp029

Masland, M. C., Lou, C., & Snowden, L. (2010). Use of communication technologies to cost-effectively increase the availability of interpretation services in healthcare settings. *Telemedicine Journal and E-Health, 16*(6), 739–745. https://doi.org/10.1089/tmj.2009.0186

McKee, M. M., Barnett, S. L., Block, R. C., & Pearson, T. A. (2011). Impact of communication on preventive services among deaf American language users. *American Journal of Preventive Medicine, 41*(1), 75–79. https://doi.org/10.1016/j.amepre.2011.03.004

McLeod, R. P., & Bently, P. C. (1996). Understanding deafness as a culture with a unique language and not a disability. *Advanced Practice Nursing Quarterly, 2*(2), 50–58.

Meador, H. E., & Zazove, P. (2005). Health care interactions with deaf culture. *Journal of the American Board of Family Medicine, 18*(3), 218–222. https://doi.org/10.3122/jabfm.18.3.218

Mitchell, R. E., & Karchmer, M. A. (2004). Chasing the mythical ten percent: Parental hearing status of deaf and hard of hearing students in the United States. *Sign Language Studies, 4*(2), 138–163. https://doi.org/10.1353/sls.2004.000510.1353/sls.2004.0005

National Association of the Deaf. (2018). *Minimum standards for video remote interpreting services in medical settings*. https://www.nad.org/about-us/position-statements/minimum-standards-for-video-remote-interpreting-services-in-medical-settings/

National Association of the Deaf. (2021). *What is the difference between a person who is "deaf," "Deaf," or "hard of hearing"?* https://www.nad.org/resources/american-sign-language/community-and-culture-frequently-asked-questions/

National Center on Disability and Journalism. (2018). *Disability language style guide*. https://ncdj.org/style-guide/

National Consortium of Interpreter Education Center. (2014). *Deaf interpreter*. http://www.interpretereducation.org/specialization/deaf-interpreter/

National Institute on Deafness and Other Communication Disorders. (2017). *Hearing aids*. https://www.nidcd.nih.gov/health/hearing-aids

National Institute on Deafness and Other Communication Disorders. (2019a). *American sign language*. https://www.nidcd.nih.gov/health/american-sign-language

National Institute on Deafness and Other Communication Disorders. (2019b). *Assistive devices for people with hearing, voice, speech, or language disorders*. https://www.nidcd.nih.gov/health/assistive-devices-people-hearing-voice-speech-or-language-disorders

National Institute on Deafness and Other Communication Disorders. (2020). Adult hearing health care. https://www.nidcd.nih.gov/health/hearing-ear-infections-deafness/adult-hearing-health-care

Oliver, M. (1996). The social model in context. In M. Oliver (Ed.), *Understanding disability from theory to practice* (1st ed., pp. 30–41). St. Martin's Press.

Oregon Health & Science University. (2021). *Inclusive language guide*. https://www.ohsu.edu/sites/default/files/2021-03/OHSU%20Inclusive%20Language%20Guide_031521.pdf

Padden, C., & Humphries, T. (1988). *Deaf in America: Voices from a culture*. Harvard University Press.

Rembis, M. A. (2010). Yes we can change: Disability studies—Enabling equality. *Journal of Postsecondary Education and Disability, 23*(1), 19–27. https://files.eric.ed.gov/fulltext/EJ888641.pdf

Rosenblum, H. A. (2015, June 22). *SHARE: Ask Howard anything* [Video]. YouTube. https://www.youtube.com/watch?v=Uy-9Iz-8xjw

Saxton, M., Havercamp, S., Wong, A., Many, G., & Schallehn, J. (2011). *Access to Medical Care.* World Institute of Disability. https://wid.org/wp-content/uploads/2016/01/access-to-medical-care-curriculum-pdf-format.pdf

Sins Invalid. (2017). *10 principles of disability justice.* https://www.sinsinvalid.org/blog/10-principles-of-disability-justice, https://static1.squarespace.com/static/5bed3674f8370ad8c02efd9a/t/5f1f0783916d8a179c46126d/1595869064521/10_Principles_of_DJ-2ndEd.pdf

Snow, K. (2016). *People first language.* Disability is Natural! https://www.disabilityisnatural.com/pfl-articles.html

Steinberg, A. G., Wiggins, E. A., Barmada, C. H., & Sullivan, V. J. (2002). Deaf women: Experiences and perceptions of healthcare system access. *Journal of Women's Health, 11*(8), 729–741. https://doi.org/10.1089/15409990260363689

Truman, A. (2020, May 2). *Why can't they just read my lips?"* https://ltclanguagesolutions.com/blog/why-cant-they-just-read-my-lips/

US Department of Justice. (2020). *A guide to disability rights law.* https://www.ada.gov/cguide.htm

Wilkinson, L. (2003). Advancing a perspective on the intersections of diversity: Challenges for research and social policy. *Canadian Ethnic Studies Journal, 35*(3), 26–38.

Womble, L., & Jones, E. (2005). *An act to provide compensation to the persons sterilized through the state's eugenic sterilization.* Encyclopedia. https://www.encyclopedia.com/history/legal-and-political-magazines/act-provide-compensation-persons-sterilized-through-states-eugenic-sterilization

Yabe, M. (2019). *Healthcare providers' and deaf patients' perspectives on video remote interpreting: A mixed methods study* [Doctoral dissertation, University of Illinois at Chicago]. University Library. http://hdl.handle.net/10027/23667.

Chapter 2
What Is an Ecology of Health Communication?

The idea of the Ecology of Health Communication came to mind after a conversation with my editor. My editor read my dissertation and told me, "Everything you explain in this paper leads to a discussion about how the readers, scholars, and researchers in the Rhetoric of Health and Medicine can work to establish an 'ecology of communication' in a health-care setting that leads to a productive exchange." Since that conversation, I sought a way to write snd define the truth of this theory, and the opprotunity came to me.

2.1 Introduction

When I interviewed deaf and hard of hearing (D/HH) patients and healthcare professionals about their experiences with video remote interpreting (VRI) versus in-person interpreters, I assumed that there were a multitude of factors that influenced their preferences, ranging from cultural to technological. Since interpreting preferences for critical and non-critical care (including their healthcare communication outcomes) are nuanced and dependent on many different cultural and physical conditions, a model of communication that examines these events must consider the broader ecology.

My editor introduced me to Margaret Syverson's (1999) book *The Wealthy of Reality: An Ecology of Composition.* In the book, Syversone discusses the ecologies of composition and presents the ecological matrix as a model for analysis, which consists of five analytical dimensions: physical-material, spatial, psychological, social, and temporal. Furthermore, Edbauer (2005) states that ecology focuses on the relations between organisms and their environment, while rhetorical ecology determines how words interact with their environments. Jensen (2015) explains that rhetorical ecology includes two modes of engagement: a flow of circulation model that traces the communication of ideas and a percolation model that draws connections between health rhetoric in historical periods.

Throughout my investigation of the Rhetoric of Health and Medicine (Meloncon & Scott, 2018), I found that the circulation model of rhetorical ecology has been

Fig. 2.1 Five analytical
dimensions of the ecology
of health communication.
Note. The central circle of
patient–provider
communication is
influenced by five
surrounding circles:
physical-material, spatial,
psychological, social, and
temporal dimensions

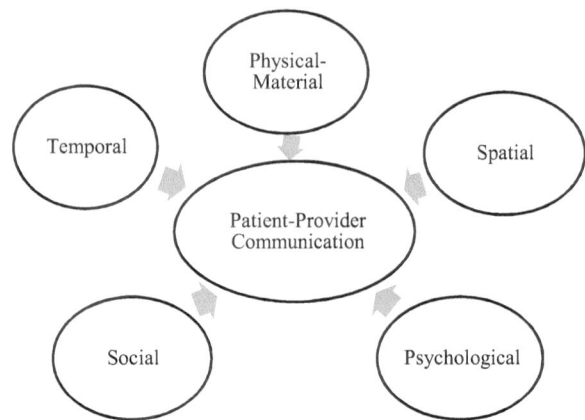

used in science and health communication. For instance, Hausman et al. (2014) and
Lawrence et al. (2014) each use the rhetorical ecology approach to identify what
factors influence the refusal of the flu vaccine, to understand patients' perspectives
on vaccinations, and to examine how to improve patient–provider communication
about vaccinations. Gonzales and Bloom-Pojar (2018) advocate the flow of medical
interpretation among healthcare providers, limited English proficiency patients, and
interpreters. However, previous research has not discussed communication practices between healthcare professionals and D/HH patients using rhetorical ecology.

Therefore, I adapted Syverson's ecological matrix. This idea led me to develop a
new theoretical framework tailored to the study of Deaf healthcare experiences,
which I call the Ecology of Health Communication (EHC). The EHC model provides insights into the specific issues of D/HH patients and their communication
with healthcare professionals (see Fig. 2.1).

2.2   Ecology of Health Communication

I also adopted a grounded theory approach to discover and construct a theory from
qualitative findings (Charmaz, 2014; Cho & Lee, 2014). Since I was determined to
let the experiences of D/HH patients and healthcare professionals speak through
this theory, I developed the EHC model with five main themes: *Physical-Material,
Spatial, Psychological, Social,* and *Temporal* (see Table 2.1).

2.3   The Dimensions of Complex Systems

Tables 2.2. and 2.3 present the characteristics of the eight D/HH patients and eight
healthcare professionals who participated in this research, respectively. Both the D/
HH patients and healthcare professionals were from the Midwestern United States

Table 2.1 Definition of the ecology of health communication

Dimension	Definition
Physical-material	Healthcare professionals' and D/HH patients' physical interactions using VRI versus in-person interpreting
Spatial	An invisible bounded space constructed across VRI versus in-person interpreting
Psychological	Healthcare professionals' and D/HH patients' mental and emotional reactions to the use of VRI versus in-person interpreting
Social	A broad range of social structures impacting the healthcare communication outcomes with VRI versus in-person interpreting
Temporal	Represents timing in the use of VRI versus in-person interpreting, and the process of interacting with D/HH patients

Table 2.2 Demographics of the deaf and hard of hearing patients

ID	Gender	Age	Primary communication	Hearing loss
BU	Male	70	ASL	Profound
DE	Female	54	ASL/PSE	Severe
ED	Female	50	ASL	Profound
IK	Female	53	ASL	Profound
JA	Male	45	ASL	Profound
ML	Female	48	ASL	Profound
RM	Male	61	ASL	Severe
RP	Male	30	ASL	Severe

Note. All IDs are coded with fictitious initials, *ASL* American Sign Language, *PSE* Pidgin Signed English
Severe = Severe Hearing Loss (61–90 dB), Profound = Profound Hearing loss (90–120 dB)

Table 2.3 Demographics of the healthcare professionals

ID	Gender	Age	Profession	Specialization
BE	Female	58	Physical therapist	Physical medicine and rehabilitation
EP	Female	31	Speech-language pathologist	Otolaryngology
GJ	Female	31	Dentist	Dentistry
GO	Female	32	Physical therapist	Physical medicine and rehabilitation
MN	Female	38	Nurse practitioner	Emergency medicine
KS	Male	26	Oral surgeon	Dentistry
TY	Female	27	Nurse practitioner	Obstetrics and gynecology
WD	Male	50	Physician	Orthopedic surgery

Note. All IDs are coded with fictitious initials

and have had experience with VRI and in-person interpreting services in medical settings over the past 10 years (Yabe, 2019).

I provide more details of their experiences in Chap. 3 (Deaf Patients' Perspectives) and Chap. 4 (Healthcare Professionals' Perspectives). In this chapter, I discuss how the EHC model can be used to better understand the five dimensions that influence patient–provider communication.

2.4   The Physical-Material Dimension

The physical-material dimension refers to healthcare professionals' and D/HH patients' physical interactions, including those involving the use of VRI screens that are too small to see the remote interpreter. This can increase the risk of mistranslations and mistreatment outcomes. Conversely, a large screen may increase the lack of privacy. For example, a large screen used during a deaf female patient's prenatal group B strep test resulted in her refusing to use a VRI interpreter. Meanwhile, an in-person interpreter can accommodate and fully access patient–provider communication without encountering such VRI technology issues.

2.4.1   Deaf and Hard of Hearing Patients

Among the D/HH patients, ED and ML reported positive physical impacts regarding the use of VRI use. However, they had been lucky in that the connectivity was good, the screen was clear, and the VRI interpreter was professional. In contrast, DE, JA, ML, RM, and BU reported negative physical impacts due to limited placement, positioning, and visual access of the screen. For example, the VRI device was limited in flexibility and screen size, which made it difficult to see the healthcare professional and the VRI interpreter on the screen. ML stated that she had to constantly and awkwardly move the screen so that she could see both the healthcare professional and the VRI interpreter. She also mentioned that an in-person interpreter must leave when a healthcare professional exits the room, but a VRI interpreter does not follow this directive.

These patients also explained that if they had had an in-person interpreter, then they could have adjusted their positions and interpreted even when the patients were placed facedown, allowing them to see the interpreter. However, since the VRI interpreter had limited mobility as far as the screen being adjusted and its position lowered, the patient was unable to see the interpreter. As a result, they missed detailed instructions such as "Please hold your breath." Having no access to such instructions made them feel invisible during treatments. These examples show how the physical-material dimension can negatively impact treatment outcomes.

2.4.2   Healthcare Professionals

The majority of the healthcare professionals raised logistical and technological issues regarding the use of VRI, due to its physical-material limitations. Among them, GJ and KS used a VRI service on a tablet, which was not mounted to anything and was movable. In this case, GJ had to ask her patients to hold the tablet, since she could not hold it while performing dental care. The tablet was also difficult for GJ to hear due to the weak volume of the speaker and microphone as well as the background noise.

What was even more disruptive was that she could not remain on the line with the same VRI interpreter, which resulted in 5 min of silence. Further supporting the conditional nature of these interpreting choices, KS was not comfortable using VRI during oral surgery.

In another instance, TY used a VRI interpreter displayed on a computer screen that was mounted in a doctor's office and not movable. The device also had a weak microphone and speaker, and there was no private space for the patients during gynecological exams. Moreover, her patients had declined to use a VRI interpreter because they were not comfortable with the lack of privacy, and they communicated this to TY in writing during the appointments. Thus, VRI was performed via a tablet since it is movable compared to a fixed computer mounted in a single room.

This is a clear example of communication being impacted by the physical-material dimension. In this regard, the use of technology can negatively affect both the human relationship outcome and the communication outcome between healthcare professionals and D/HH patients.

2.5 The Spatial Dimension

VRI and in-person interpreting are constructed across an invisible space. For example, a VRI interpreter may lack a human trust relationship with the patient, while in-person interpreters can easily develop this relationship between healthcare professionals and patients. However, VRI has spatial limitations, such as during physical or dental surgery, or when a patient is lying in a hospital bed. Conversely, an in-person interpreter has the spatial flexibility to accommodate a D/HH patient so that he/she can see both the interpreter and the healthcare professional, while the interpreter can see the patient's condition and provide accurate translations. In this case, the boundaries of the relationships and communication depend on the type of interpreting service and the spaces occupied during treatment.

2.5.1 Deaf and Hard of Hearing Patients

Communication in the spatial dimension plays an important role in the relationship between D/HH patients and healthcare professionals. For example, DE pointed out that VRI interpreters struggled to build a human trust relationship and could only provide limited access to facial and body language, compared to in-person interpreters. In other instances, BU, DE, ED, RP, and RM experienced poor connectivity, which caused lag-delays for translations during treatments. In contrast, BU, DE, IK, RM, ED, and RP preferred in-person interpreting services for critical care, since such interpreters allowed for extensive spatial access for patient–provider communication such as clarifying information regarding diagnosis, treatment, and surgery/hospitalization, and assessing the patient's language.

In regard to the latter, BU, DE, and RP mentioned that in-person interpreters were able to assess and accommodate their language levels. It should be noted that BU works as a certified deaf interpreter (CDI). A CDI is a specialist who provides interpreting, translation, and transliteration services, utilizing ASL and other visual and tactile signing forms used by individuals who are Deaf, hard of hearing, and Deaf-Blind (National Consortium of Interpreter Education Center, 2014). However, BU argued that the VRI interpreter was unable to accommodate D/HH patients with limited literacy skills. He has translated for D/HH patients, and he has seen patients become very frustrated when the communication is unsuccessful, not only for D/HH patients from English-speaking countries, but also those from non-English-speaking countries. Additionally, he explained that if the patients had some cognitive disabilities or were not fluent in sign language, then they might need accommodations for not only treatments but also for registration.

DE agreed:

> I think an in-person interpreter is best because the interpreter can then, kind of, make an assessment about the patients' sign style and skills, maybe even their intellectual level. They can be a better match for the patients' needs.

2.5.2 Healthcare Professionals

Among the healthcare professionals, EP believed that the VRI screen and the slight delay in transmission diminished the interpersonal relationship between providers and patients. She has dealt with patients with cognitive impairment after a stroke or brain surgery, or other language barriers. In-person interpreting provided more effective communication for cognitive and speech therapy and for family meetings.

GJ, KS, and WD preferred in-person interpreters for critical care due to the demands of surgical care. Additionally, they not only preferred them for effective communication for critical care, but also for the flexibility of translation in different spatial dimensions. KS explained that in-person interpreting was beneficial for having an interaction in the waiting room and talking directly to a patient. Both GO and KS expressed that in-person interpreting increased the trust between the patient and provider, which led to better possibilities of successful and compliant treatment. GO often places her patients in different positions, such as facedown, during physical therapy. In-person interpreters were able to accommodate the physical movement, in contrast to VRI, which was limited in this respect.

BE discussed how VRI is limited in the spatial dimension:

> Sometimes using the VRI is difficult in a noisy area like a gym. It is hard for the interpreter and therapist [and patient if it is a language issue] to hear one another. It is much better in a private room, but they are not always available.

In this regard, spaces with noisy backgrounds can make it difficult for a VRI interpreter to access all the information from a group discussion with the healthcare professional, the patient, and the patient's family. This situation negatively affects the psychological dimension. Thus, invisible qualities of the spatial dimension, such as interpersonal connections, can impact patient–provider communication and treatment outcomes.

2.6   The Psychological Dimension

The psychological dimension includes the times when D/HH patients are assigned (without notification) VRI interpreters instead of in-person interpreters. Consequently, they become disappointed and/or angry during their treatments. Meanwhile, healthcare professionals may grow irritated because they are unable to fully communicate due to the poor connectivity of VRI and the time pressure from consecutive appointments with other patients. These factors negatively impact patient–provider communication, treatment outcomes, and healthcare experiences.

2.6.1   Deaf and Hard of Hearing Patients

Concerning the psychological dimension, DE, ED, and IK expressed that there was no emotional connection between the patient and provider when using VRI interpreters. DE stated,

> If it is a real live interpreter, then I can really get that rapport and have that connection. With VRI, since it is almost too neutral, I do not get a chance to really form a connection.

The psychological dimension also impacts communication in regard to another concern: miscommunication between healthcare professionals and D/HH patients. BU, DE, and JA were assigned VRI interpreters without being notified beforehand. Additionally, IK, who was being treated for breast cancer, was not comfortable using a VRI interpreter due to poor connectivity and the lack of a human relationship between the physician and herself. Yet, hospitals are unaware of such issues. ED sadly expressed,

> Unfortunately, hospitals in the area, you know, doctors or nurses and things like that, are not understanding in two ways. First, they do not understand how to use VRI. I have seen this happen so many times. They struggle with the equipment, or they put it in the wrong place. Sometimes, they try to give it me. However, I cannot sign and hold the iPad at the same time. There are also some situations where VRI is just not appropriate such as a traumatic mental health situation, news of a death, a serious diagnosis, or if there are various tests/ procedures in which the patients cannot sit and sign because they have to maneuver around the room. I think that there are lots of people who do not understand the law and what it really means.

In this regard, sensitive topics or critical treatments performed with VRI interpreters can negatively impact patient–provider communication, human relationships, and treatment outcomes. Moreover, it can lead to possible negative consequences for patients, who might be less likely to return for additional treatments or be open with their providers. Meanwhile, the healthcare providers might feel uncomfortable using VRI interpreters due to the various issues regarding the technology. In contrast to VRI, in-person interpreting positively increases translation accuracy, enhances the creation of a human relationship, and improves the outcomes of critical treatments. Thus, it is important to consider these potential impacts on the psychological dimension.

2.6.2 Healthcare Professionals

Among the healthcare professionals, GJ and KS mentioned the negative effects that VRI had on their relationships with patients. GJ preferred in-person interpreting during dental procedures because patients do not generally feel comfortable in a dentist's office. With VRI, then technical issues could arise such as poor connectivity, small screen size, and limited mobility, which might make the patients feel more uncomfortable. Having an in-person interpreter can help avoid these issues and improve the human relationship between the provider and patient. GJ explained,

> I think you just lose something when you cannot see [the interpreter] in person. There is some kind of emotional disconnection, so it makes it a little bit harder.

KS had experiences with a VRI interpreter's lack of professionalism. Specifically, when his patient required a tooth extraction, the interpreter interrupted and stated that more treatment options should be provided. The interpreter's opinion had a negative influence on KS's interaction with his patient and his patient's decision-making. Hence, the communication outcomes of the psychological dimension are closely associated with the physical-material and spatial dimensions.

2.7 The Social Dimension

The social dimension encompasses a broad range of social structures. One example is when a hospital administrator makes a budget-related decision to cut the number of in-person interpreters and increase the number of VRI interpreters. Such a decision then negatively impacts the quality of medical interpreting services as a whole. Meanwhile, the recent coronavirus outbreak has increased the popularity of VRI. This has raised new issues for patient–provider communication and the demands for training needs, due to the general lack of instruction on cultural interactions with D/HH patients.

2.7.1 Deaf and Hard of Hearing Patients

The use of VRI by hospital administration systems has impacted the quality of medical interpreting services, which, in turn, has negatively affected D/HH patients' psychological dimensions. IK shared her complaint concerning the unavailability of in-person interpreters because VRI interpreters were already available. ED was concerned that hospitals and providers did not recognize the importance of the legal obligations related to communication with patients. Additionally, RP argued that VRI interpreters generally lack medical training. He also pointed out that a clinic should determine how often it uses VRI versus in-person interpreting services (based on specific treatment needs) when making decisions about investing in such services. RP stated,

> Most of the VRI interpreters are not really medically trained, or not focused on medical technology. Sometimes they do not know the terminology...My mom is a nurse, and she told me that they ordered [VRI] equipment for two million dollars, but they have only used it once or twice in five years.

2.7.2 Healthcare Professionals

The healthcare professionals also noted how a hospital administration's budget can affect the quality of interpreting services. BE and WD (who both managed a clinic and directly administered the budgets) were concerned about the loss of funds if a patient failed to show up for an appointment, as the clinic cannot request a refund from them. Thus, the use of VRI on demand could help the facility avoid financial losses.

However, BE, GJ, and WD pointed out the benefits of using in-person interpreting even if it is expensive. BE explained that she would use an in-person interpreter for a specific patient with cognitive disabilities because her patient has difficulty understanding VRI translation. Hence, she would choose the interpreting modality based on the type of patient, communication effectiveness, and treatment outcomes.

Furthermore, EP and GJ pointed out the lack of medical training for VRI. In this regard, both of them received no training before they used VRI for the first time. Through the lens of the social dimension, hospital administration systems are impacted by VRI, in-person interpreter availability, and training availability, which, in turn, influence patient–provider communication outcomes.

2.8 The Temporal Dimension

The temporal dimension refers to finding the right time to use a specific service. For instance, although healthcare professionals and D/HH patients may prefer to use in-person interpreting for emergency care, they may end up using VRI interpreters during such times due to the immediacy of the situation. The temporal dimension also concerns life experiences in which healthcare professionals have been trained to communicate with D/HH patients and have become comfortable treating D/HH patients with an interpreter.

2.8.1 Deaf and Hard of Hearing Patients

Timing is essential in securing an interpreter for critical care versus non-critical care because it impacts the patient–provider communication outcome. The temporal dimension is often associated with the psychological and social dimensions.

The majority of the D/HH patients pointed out that VRI had a positive impact on the temporal dimension, citing specific reasons. For instance, BU had surgery and waited for in-person interpreters all day. In this case, he would have preferred a VRI interpreter when several doctors came to check on him. RP preferred in-person interpreters, but he would use a VRI interpreter if no in-person interpreter were available, or if there were no time to wait for an in-person interpreter, such as in emergency care. DE and ED reported that they would not mind using VRI for emergency care, at least until an in-person interpreter became available. However, BU and ED stated that VRI was time-consuming to set up, due to the poor connectivity.

From another perspective, DE, ED, IK, JA, ML, RM, and RP observed how in-person interpreting positively influences patient–provider communication compared to VRI. For example, ML had an in-person interpreter who stayed with her the whole time during her child's birth. If interpreting had been performed through VRI, then it would have been impossible to stay online during the extended care that she received all day.

2.8.2 Healthcare Professionals

According to the healthcare professionals, timing is essential in terms of treatment outcomes. For instance, MN preferred to use in-person interpreting for urgent care, but securing an interpreter required several hours' notice. Due to these time constraints, she used VRI for communication accommodations. Additionally, it was difficult to find an in-person interpreter during odd hours, since the hospital did not have a contract for providing in-person interpreters overnight.

Among the other healthcare professionals, EP, WD, GO, and GJ agreed that it was convenient to use VRI. EP pointed out that it was unrealistic to have an in-person interpreter come to the hospital for a patient's emergency care, while GO stated that VRI was already available in her clinic. Moreover, TY mentioned that her clinic did not have in-person interpreters and depended on VRI or family interpreters. Therefore, it can be stated that VRI has a positive impact on the temporal dimension for emergency care or when in-person interpreters are unavailable, which ensures efficient patient–provider communication.

2.9 Conclusion

2.9.1 Comparison Between Deaf and Hard of Hearing Patients and Healthcare Professionals

The analysis of the EHC model suggests that D/HH patients and healthcare professionals had similar experiences with VRI technology issues, such as the physical-material dimension, and they recommended improving VRI equipment. Also, both groups noted positive aspects of in-person interpreting such as effective patient–provider communication, stronger patient–provider relationships, and full access to communication in the spatial dimension.

For the D/HH patients, in-person interpreting allowed for better healthcare experiences, while the healthcare professionals found that in-person interpreting allowed them to provide better quality treatments. Both groups experienced VRI as generating negative emotional and mental reactions during medical procedures in the psychological dimension.

However, the two groups had different perspectives on the social dimension. First, the D/HH patients considered VRI a waste of money, while the healthcare professionals asserted that VRI saves money for the hospital or clinic. Second, both the D/HH patients and healthcare professionals were concerned about the lack of VRI training for healthcare practitioners. Third, while the D/HH patients would accept the use of VRI for emergency care until an in-person interpreter arrived, the healthcare professionals would prefer to use VRI for emergency care, due to time constraints.

Overall, the ECH model allowed us to identify how the five analytical dimensions affect patient–provider communication, treatment outcomes, and healthcare experiences. Moreover, in-person interpreting is qualitatively better for healthcare communication access. Therefore, healthcare professionals should be prepared to prioritize what D/HH patients prefer, which is in-person interpreting.

References

Charmaz, K. (2014). *Constructing grounded theory*. SAGE.

Cho, J. Y., & Lee, E. (2014). Reducing confusion about grounded theory and qualitative content analysis: Similarities and differences. *Qualitative Report, 19*(32), 1–20. https://doi.org/10.46743/2160-3715/2014.1028

Edbauer, J. (2005). Unframing models of public distribution: From rhetorical situation to rhetorical ecologies. *Rhetoric Society Quarterly, 35*(4), 5–24. https://doi.org/10.1080/02773940509391320

Gonzales, L., & Bloom-Pojar, R. (2018). A dialogue with medical interpreters about rhetoric, culture, and language. *Rhetoric of Health and Medicine, 1*(1–2), 193–212. https://doi.org/10.5744/rhm.2018.1002

Hausman, B. L., Ghebremichael, M., Hayek, P., & Mack, E. (2014). 'Poisonous, filthy, loathsome, damnable stuff': The rhetorical ecology of vaccination concern. *Yale Journal of Biology and Medicine, 87*(4), 403–416. http://www.ncbi.nlm.nih.gov/pmc/articles/pmc4257028/

Jensen, R. E. (2015). An ecological turn in rhetoric of health scholarship: Attending to the historical flow and percolation of ideas, assumptions, and arguments. *Communication Quarterly, 63*(5), 522–526. https://doi.org/10.1080/01463373.2015.1103600

Lawrence, H. Y., Hausman, B. L., & Dannenberg, C. J. (2014). Reframing medicine's publics: The local as a public of vaccine refusal. *Journal of Medical Humanities, 35*(2), 111–129. https://doi.org/10.1007/s10912-014-9278-4

Meloncon, L., & Scott, J. B. (Eds.). (2018). *Methodologies for the rhetoric of health and medicine.* Routledge.

National Consortium of Interpreter Education Center. (2014). *Deaf interpreter.* http://www.interpretereducation.org/specialization/deaf-interpreter/

Syverson, M. (1999). *The wealth of reality: An ecology of composition.* Southern Illinois University Press.

Yabe, M. (2019). *Healthcare providers' and deaf patients' perspectives on video remote interpreting: A mixed methods study* [Doctoral dissertation, University of Illinois Chicago]. University Library. http://hdl.handle.net/10027/23667

Chapter 3
Deaf and Hard of Hearing Patients' Perspectives

Well, my parents are deaf, and my mother had to go to a cardiologist. For several years, they provided an interpreter, and everything was seamless. Then all of the sudden, they used a VRI, and my mother was in shock. She had never used one before. Previously, she had a relationship in which she used to be able to communicate and joke with the doctor. Now, that relationship is gone because they wheeled in a VRI. Then, she was gone.—DE, a Deaf Patient

3.1 Introduction

The narrative above is from one of the deaf and hard of hearing (D/HH) patients. When I developed a pilot Disability Studies curriculum for the College of Medicine at the University of Illinois, Chicago, I received feedback from the medical students that they wanted to learn more about the voices of patients with disabilities. They asked me why issues such as positioning are important for D/HH patients. Accordingly, I explained that American Sign Language (ASL) communication requires clear sight. When using video remote interpreting (VRI), the D/HH patients have to face the VRI interpreter on the computer or iPad screen, preventing them from looking at the doctor and reading the doctor's facial expressions. The small screen size also demands focused visual attention, which limits opportunities for the D/HH signers to read the room and access additional information.

Meanwhile, more subtle changes and information that can be tracked in the three-dimensional world are flattened or erased on VRI. All of these dimensions directly impact language access and affective experiences. Through my research, I was struck by how frequently these D/HH patients expressed shock, distrust, and vulnerability in the context of VRI, and how using in-person interpreters was far less stressful. Their stories reminded me of my own healthcare experiences as a deaf patient. Hence, I decided to write out the narratives from eight D/HH patients whom I interviewed. To protect their anonymity, the patients' names were coded with

---

To protect the anonymity of the patients featured in this chapter, their names were coded with fictitious initials.

M. Yabe, *Deaf Rhetoric*, SpringerBriefs in Public Health,
https://doi.org/10.1007/978-3-030-96245-6_3

fictitious initials, i.e., BU, DE, ED, IK, JA, ML, RM, and RP. All the patients had used VRI at hospitals or clinics in the Midwestern United States (Yabe, 2019).

Finally, I want to note that their stories sometimes overlap with Chap. 2 (What is an Ecology of Health Communication?). However, Chap. 2 discusses the D/HH patients' stories through the lens of the Ecology of Health Communication model, while Chap. 3 discusses their stories through the lens of the whole human.

3.2 Deaf and Hard of Hearing Patients' Narratives

3.2.1 BU

BU is a 70-year-old man with profound hearing loss. He uses ASL as his primary means of communication. His first experience with VRI was not good. When he visited a surgeon at his office, BU had an in-person interpreter. Then, as he waited for another interpreter at the next appointment, he did not know that the interpretation would take place via a VRI device. He thought that the VRI screen was a blood pressure machine, and he continued waiting for an in-person interpreter. When he learned that this machine was a VRI device, he was shocked. He was not prepared to use it because he had assumed that he would have an in-person interpreter. During the appointment, he had to frequently look back and forth between his doctor and the VRI interpreter. Consequently, he had to stop using the interpreter in that way and asked that the screen be moved so that he could simultaneously see the doctor and the VRI interpreter.

He also experienced problems with poor connectivity, small screen size, and limited placement, which made the VRI device insufficient in allowing for patient–provider communication. Ironically, he saw that the same interpreter on the VRI call had been his in-person interpreter:

> It was the same interpreter from another facility, but I did not understand why. If I was see-ing the same interpreter on VRI as the one in person, then why don't they just use the one in person all the time?

BU explained that he would prefer to use VRI for a short medical visit, due to sched-ule conflicts or time constraints, instead of waiting for an in-person interpreter. However, when he was receiving critical treatment in an intensive care unit, his doctors came to check on him. Since he could not write (due to his physical condi-tion), he preferred to use VRI rather than waiting all day for an in-person interpreter.

BU also suggested VRI training for new patients as well as for healthcare profes-sionals in operating the equipment. Moreover, he emphasized the importance of patient–provider communication and education for medical students and medical schools. He clarified that VRI is appropriate in the emergency room, due to time demands, but in-person interpreting is more beneficial for pre-arranged appoint-ments. Finally, BU recommended improving VRI equipment for better connectivity by using a specific network that can accommodate VRI services.

3.2.2   DE

DE is a 54-year-old female with severe hearing loss. She uses ASL and Pidgin Sign English as her primary forms of communication. Her first experience with VRI was not positive. When she and her hearing daughter visited the hospital, the doctor set up the VRI device. However, due to the poor placement of the VRI machine, she felt awkward using it because she had to sign to the VRI interpreter while the doctor stood behind her. Her second experience with VRI was a biopsy after a mammogram. The treatment was in the basement of the hospital, where the network access was poor. She noted,

> Everyone looked so excited, calling it a wonderful innovation. Although I did not agree with their assumption, I accepted it anyway. Then, they opened the laptop and explained the procedure. However, since the doctor was speaking from behind me, I had to frequently turn around to communicate. It was just very awkward.

> Then, after they closed the laptop and sent the video interpreter away, there I was, lying on the table without an interpreter. At that time, I did not know what they were doing, since there was no communication.

Interestingly, DE had been assigned an in-person interpreter at the same hospital several years earlier. However, at the later procedure, the hospital did not inform her that requesting an interpreter meant receiving VRI. In general, she preferred using an in-person interpreter for both critical and non-critical care because she could see their facial expressions and establish a rapport and connection. Yet, she mentioned that she would not mind using VRI for an emergency until an in-person interpreter arrived at the hospital within a few hours. Meanwhile, she would not accept VRI for a pre-arranged appointment.

DE also offered several suggestions for improving VRI services: training VRI interpreters to explain to healthcare professionals how to use VRI and raising doctors' awareness not to stand behind the D/HH patient. As for the latter, the doctor should stand in front of or next to the computer so that the D/HH patient can see both the doctor and the interpreter. Moreover, VRI interpreters should advocate on behalf of D/HH patients. Specifically, D/HH patients have the right to choose their interpreting preferences, but many patients may not be aware of their rights. As a result, they are left to advocate for themselves.

3.2.3   ED

ED is a 50-year-old female with profound hearing loss. She uses ASL as her primary means of communication and is working on obtaining a certified deaf interpreter license. Her first experience with VRI was positive. When she had VRI for a follow-up appointment, the connectivity was good, the screen was clear, and she was able to understand the VRI interpreter. However, when she had VRI a second time, her nurse struggled with using the machine and connecting to the VRI interpreter. ED became tired of waiting, so she told the nurse to forget the VRI and go ahead and write back and forth, since it was only a follow-up appointment.

ED also mentioned that she would not like to use VRI for a critical procedure such as surgery or something that needs to be discussed in-depth (e.g., test results). She believed that VRI is appropriate for follow-up appointments and simple tests. Additionally, she would only accept VRI until an in-person interpreter could arrive at the hospital. However, she would not be willing to use it if the hospital only requested VRI and did not check the availability of an in-person interpreter.

Moreover, ED found that hospitals do not understand three issues regarding interpreters. First, doctors and nurses may not know how to use VRI and struggle with the equipment. For example, they place it in the wrong location, or they ask D/HH patients to hold the iPad, even though the patients cannot sign and hold the iPad at the same time. Second, they inappropriately provide VRI for mental health care, news of a death, or serious results of various tests/procedures in a room where the patients cannot sit and sign, since they would have to maneuver around to see the VRI. Third, they often assume that providing VRI satisfies the requirements of the Americans with Disabilities Act (ADA). ED unhappily remarked,

> They think that the communication is clear and that the patient clearly understands everything. However, sometimes, there is a big misunderstanding. The doctor does not realize the importance of clear communication. If the patients do not understand the diagnosis, then how can they properly take the prescribed medicines? This will eventually cause problems, which is sad.

3.2.4   IK

IK is a 53-year-old female with profound hearing loss. She uses ASL as her primary form of communication. She has had negative experiences with VRI during her breast cancer treatments. For example, the hospital provided an in-person interpreter for her treatments, but in some instances, they had no choice but to provide VRI when an in-person interpreter was unavailable. Due to her medication, she was unable to effectively use VRI and she had to ask the VRI interpreter to repeat the information. There was no bond and no relationship with the VRI interpreter, and she felt that using one was emotionally cold:

> I noticed that when you have an in-person interpreter, there is information that you can build upon and retain. However, with VRI, they do not necessarily understand the doctor. As a result, there is a lot of misunderstanding between myself and the interpreter. I also feel like there are different types of information being offered. The VRI process is not as effective compared to a warm-bodied interpreter.

Moreover, when IK's sons required emergency care, the hospital asked them to provide family interpreting. IK understood that this was an inappropriate request, which disturbed the care for her family. She declined and requested an on-site interpreter. She pointed out that these issues are often related to hospital systems. She suggested that doctors, nurses, schedulers, case managers, and those who coordinate appointments and interpreting services need training on how to appropriately provide interpreting services for specific procedures.

3.2.5 JA

JA is a 45-year-old male with profound hearing loss. He uses ASL as his primary form of communication. He has also had negative experiences with VRI. When he visited the emergency room with his deaf children, VRI was provided. However, he was not comfortable using it because he had to move the VRI around for himself and for his children:

> There is one impact that I feel is deleterious. It is when I feel like I sign to them and it is my kids who are basically forcing me to change the screen so they can speak and reply. In this case, you have to constantly maneuver the screen. It is a lot of physical activity that should not happen.

For many years, when JA visited the emergency room for an appointment, he promptly received an on-site interpreter. However, nowadays, he is provided with VRI. In one instance, he had to educate the hospital administrator that it was inappropriate to provide VRI unless a D/HH patient requested it and that it would not be feasible to use VRI for Deaf-Blind patients. He continued to explain the legal obligations and that if the hospital did not follow such obligations, it could lead to lawsuits. He also argued that on-site interpreters would save a lot of money over VRI. As a result, the hospital provided an in-person interpreter for his care.

JA also suggested eliminating VRI and having on-site interpreters or educating nurses to become fluent in ASL so that the hospital could save money by not hiring on-site interpreters. It would also be convenient to have a deaf nurse or other healthcare provider who is familiar with medical jargon and terminology in order to reduce the degree of misunderstanding and improve patient–provider communication. With such changes, it is possible that more D/HH patients would be willing to visit deaf-friendly clinics or hospitals.

3.2.6 ML

ML is a 48-year-old female with profound hearing loss. She uses ASL as her primary means of communication. Her experience with VRI was positive, except for the way that her doctor managed the equipment. She had good connectivity with the VRI device and was able to see and understand the VRI interpreter. However, she stated,

> The only disappointing part of it was the way that the doctor managed it. The doctor was simply looking at the interpreter, instead of looking at me.

She mentioned that interactions in patient–provider communication could be improved by explaining to providers how to appropriately use VRI and on-site interpreters. In this regard, if providers knew how to deal with VRI services, then patient–provider communication would go more smoothly. ML also suggested improving the VRI equipment (e.g., increasing the flexibility of the cord so that it can bend and mold to the iPad) so that patients can lie down and still see the VRI screen, along with better connectivity to avoid disconnections during procedures.

Meanwhile, she was willing to have either a VRI interpreter or an in-person interpreter for critical or non-critical care, and she explained the advantages and disadvantages of both interpreting services. She observed that the VRI interpreter has limited visual space on the screen, so he/she might not understand everything that occurs, whereas the in-person interpreter can leave with the doctor and access information related to the entire situation. ML provided an example of when her daughter was giving birth and the baby was premature. There was a team of approximately ten healthcare professionals in the room. In this case, having an in-person interpreter was beneficial for full access to the information. Finally, having a certified interpreter is essential because VRI companies have different quality levels of interpreters, with some lacking medical training.

3.2.7 RM

RM is a 61-year-old male with severe hearing loss. He uses ASL as his primary form of communication. His first experience with VRI was not satisfactory. When his doctor notified him that he was going to use VRI, he was willing to try it out. However, when he saw the VRI device being set up, he noted that the function of the equipment was incredibly slow due to a poor connection. There was also a lag time and delay between the initial communication and the interpretation. There were additional problems with the machine. For example, the healthcare staff could not place it at the correct angle, so it was limited for use in translation. Hence, the VRI was ineffective.

RM provided feedback to the nurses about his first-time experience with VRI. However, when he used VRI a second time, they still had the same problems. It was clear that the nurses had not considered his feedback about how to improve the equipment. Then, he went to another room in which he had to lie down on the table. In this situation, there was no way that they could manipulate the VRI device, so he did not know what they were doing. Once again, the VRI was ineffective.

In general, he felt more comfortable using in-person interpreters because they provide more precise and real-time information, and they can interact with the doctor and move around. Conversely, when using VRI, RM felt stuck waiting for the interpreters' responses, which were not very timely. He also believed that in-person interpreters would be appropriate for serious procedures and that VRI would not be acceptable in such cases:

> The VRI interpreter may not know me very well, and they may be limited in what they can see. So, they may not even know, for example, what body part is being discussed. It is also not a situation in which I can control the VRI, since they are in control of the equipment and how the interpreter interprets the information.

Moreover, RM explained that D/HH patients may struggle to find a doctor who provides in-person interpreters. He felt lucky to identify a provider who is aware of his communication needs and provides an interpreter, allowing him to access equal communication. However, sometimes it is challenging to schedule an appointment with the doctor due to the limitations of scheduling (especially for emergency care) or because an interpreter is not available. In this case, he is willing to use VRI as a last resort.

3.2.8 RP

RP is a 30-year-old male with severe hearing loss. He uses ASL as his primary means of communication and identifies himself as a hard of hearing person. If he wears his hearing aid and receives non-critical care, then he prefers no interpreters. He can speak and communicate if his doctor talks to him face-to-face, is deaf-friendly, and knows how to communicate with a D/HH patient. However, if he has no hearing aid, he prefers to call in an interpreter for both critical and non-critical procedures.

His first experience with VRI was when he did not have his hearing aid. He was shocked when he was offered VRI, and he thought it seemed kind of robotic. He also felt that the use of VRI did not go smoothly due to time lags and poor connectivity. In many instances, he had to ask the VRI interpreter to repeat herself, and they went back and forth in the same manner. When he had surgery, he was fortunate to receive two interpreters for the group meeting with his doctor and his parents, which went smoothly. His parents do not know how to sign.

RP's mother works as a nurse, and he learned from her that hospitals have spent too much money on VRI devices but rarely use them. Additionally, most VRI interpreters are not medically trained or are not focused on medical technology. Thus, the hospital should be budgeting for in-person interpreters to accommodate for appropriate treatments. He stated,

> I understand that the hospital is trying to save money, but they fail to understand that deaf people do not depend on VRI. Instead, they prefer to depend on an in-person interpreter, with face-to-face communication.

also stated that his interpreting preferences depend on the situation. For example, if the issues are surgery, hospitalization, or something serious, then he would request an in-person interpreter to ensure that everything goes smoothly. Additionally, he mentioned that he feels more comfortable asking questions and clarifying information with an in-person interpreter, since the in-person interpreter can read a patient's body language and make certain adjustments for the patient's comprehension. As for emergency care, he would accept VRI in the case of time constraints and the unavailability of in-person interpreters. However, if it was only a checkup, then he might not even request an interpreter at all.

3.3 Conclusion

3.3.1 Comparison of Experiences with Video Remote Interpreting and In-Person Interpreting

During the interviews, the D/HH patients shared their positive and negative experiences with VRI and in-person interpreting, in addition to their interpreting preferences regarding critical and non-critical care. While ED, ML, and BU had good experiences with VRI, BU, DE, ED, RP, and RM complained about VRI technology issues such as poor connectivity, limited mobility, and device placement. Moreover, BU, DE, and JA were offered VRI without being notified beforehand. This is problematic and unethical because the hospitals did not respect the D/HH patients' interpreting preferences, which resulted in unpleasant experiences.

Conversely, DE, ED, IK, JA, ML, RM, and RP expressed positive reactions to in-person interpreting because it allows for effective communication and translation accuracy. The D/HH patients also pointed out that in-person interpreters are generally better because they can understand the patients and have the ability to adjust positioning and assess the dynamics in the room, thus increasing the accuracy of communication. Only BU and IK were unable to obtain an in-person interpreter for critical care, due to limited availability.

3.3.2 Comparison of Interpreting Preferences for Critical and Non-critical Care

BU, DE, ED, and RP did not prefer VRI for critical care, but they would accept it for a specific reason such as when there is no in-person interpreter available, or if there is no time to wait for an interpreter during emergency care. Meanwhile, ED and IK believed that VRI would be appropriate for non-critical care such as follow-up visits. Yet, BU, DE, IK, RM, and RP preferred in-person interpreting for both critical and non-critical care because it increases the ease of accessing and clarifying information during a medical visit. Even if the appointments were pre-arranged, BU and DE still preferred in-person interpreting.

3.3.3 Deaf and Hard of Hearing Patients' Recommendations

All the D/HH patients provided suggestions for improving VRI services such as by enhancing connectivity, attaching a gooseneck to the rolling carts that carry the tablet, and furnishing a larger screen. They also suggested more education on interpreting for medical students and healthcare professionals, VRI interpreters, hospital administrators, and D/HH patients and their families. For instance, IK suggested that hospital administrators need more training on how to determine D/HH patients' interpreting preferences. Hospital administrators should not assume that VRI services are sufficient for accommodating D/HH patients, and they should be aware of such patients' preferences based on the different types of treatment sessions. Additionally, ED suggested that VRI companies should take their responsibilities seriously under the ADA, by educating hospitals about how to use VRI and providing resources to hospitals. More importantly, it is crucial to thoughtfully consider the feedback of D/HH patients, since they are experts on their lives and communication needs and they have the wisdom to promote better healthcare experiences.

Reference

Yabe, M. (2019). *Healthcare providers' and deaf patients' perspectives on video remote interpreting: A mixed methods study* [Doctoral dissertation, University of Illinois, Chicago]. University Library. http://hdl.handle.net/10027/23667

Chapter 4

Healthcare Professionals' Perspectives

I will say that in-person interpreting, in my experience, allows for much more person-to-person interaction between my patients and myself. And, to me, this leads to more treatment acceptance and better treatment outcomes.—KS, Oral Surgeon

4.1 Introduction

The narrative above changed my patient perspective toward healthcare professionals. Throughout my research, I learned about different perspectives from healthcare professionals, especially how they value patient–provider communication for better treatment outcomes and healthcare experiences, even if they do not have Deaf cultural knowledge. These interview experiences provided me with a new lens through which to view healthcare providers' perspectives.

Thus, I decided to present the narratives from eight healthcare professionals, since they can serve as a beneficial resource for healthcare professionals who are preparing to work with deaf and hard of hearing (D/HH) patients, limited English proficiency (LEP) patients, and medical and healthcare students who want to learn about their colleagues' experiences. In addition, their stories are beneficial for D/HH patients who want to understand healthcare professionals' perspectives.

These healthcare professionals worked in different hospitals, including public and private clinics in the Midwestern United States, and they had treated both D/HH patients and LEP patients using video remote interpreting (VRI) and in-person interpreting. To protect their anonymity, their names were coded with fictitious initials: BE, EP, GJ, GO, MN, KS, TY, and WD.

Finally, I want to note that their stories sometimes overlap with Chap. 2 (What Is an Ecology of Health Communication?). However, Chap. 2 discusses their stories through the Ecology of Health Communication model, while Chap. 4 discusses each of the healthcare professionals' stories as that of a whole human under the enforcement of the law.

To protect the anonymity of the healthcare professionals featured in this chapter, their names were coded with fictitious initials.

39
M. Yabe, *Deaf Rhetoric*, SpringerBriefs in Public Health,
https://doi.org/10.1007/978-3-030-96245-6_4

4.2 Healthcare Professionals' Narratives

4.2.1 BE

BE is a 58-year-old female who has worked as a physical therapist for 37 years. She has experience using VRI and in-person interpreters for both D/HH patients and LEP patients. She explained that there is not much difference when treating D/HH patients and LEP patients, but she emphasized the importance of patient–provider communication. Additionally, she felt that it was not an issue to use VRI for non-deaf LEP patients, as they can still hear the VRI interpreter when they lie down. However, it is not feasible to use VRI for D/HH patients because they need to see the VRI interpreter.

In some instances, when BE requested an in-person interpreter, the D/HH patients did not show up for their appointments. Since this occasionally occurs, VRI is economically practical and helpful for hospitals to avoid financial losses. BE also uses in-person interpreters for young pediatric patients because young children are unable to understand the VRI interpreter. She even had an adult Deaf patient who was cognitively challenged and unable to understand the VRI interpreter.

However, BE has never had issues with in-person interpreters because of their ability to be face-to-face with patients and mobile. This makes it easier for them to fully establish patient–provider communication. In contrast, with VRI, there is sometimes a delay in the responses to questions due to connectivity problems. Furthermore, regardless of whether VRI or an in-person interpreter is provided, BE emphasized that a professional interpreter should be offered, not a family member or friend:

> It is our mission to provide patient care and it is absolutely our responsibility to provide language services to every patient who needs it. As for professional interpretive services, it is really clear in all of the hospital policies that we should not be using family or friends to interpret.

4.2.2 EP

EP is a 31-year-old female who has worked as a speech-language pathologist for eight years. Specifically, she works with brain injury and stroke patients, and she has also worked with D/HH patients using both VRI and in-person interpreting services. When she worked in a large hospital, VRI was set up in emergency rooms and intensive care units. When she first saw a VRI in an intensive care unit, she had no training and no understanding of how to use it. Even so, she thought that it was convenient and helpful, though the hospital had not offered formal training in its use.

EP had used VRI when she treated a Deaf patient who used American Sign Language (ASL) and had suffered a stroke. She noticed that the patient had a language barrier even with VRI and believed that an in-person interpreter would have been more appropriate for the patient's communication needs.

Overall, EP prefers in-person interpreters for cognitive therapy and speech-language therapy because it is helpful for developing interpersonal connections, covering sensitive topics with subtle language dynamics, and holding group meetings with patients' families.

EP also pointed out the challenges of communication with hard of hearing patients, which differs from that with Deaf patients. Hard of hearing patients are non-signers who depend on reading lips. Hence, they have difficulty understanding their doctors who may wear masks and take certain health precautions in a hospital room. Additionally, EP felt that training could help improve patient–provider communication.

> I feel like the education is varied, and there are such diverse and different medical, hospital, and patient interactions. I think that it would be helpful for medical students to have some idea about how to effectively communicate with patients.

4.2.3   GJ

GJ is a 31-year-old female who has worked as a dentist for three years. She shared her experiences in a previous workplace, where one of the other dentists was fluent in ASL. Since D/HH patients came to see the dentist, GJ also learned a little ASL. She once treated a deaf patient and her son. When she first met them, she did not know about their language needs, so she simply wrote back and forth for the first appointment. Then, she ordered VRI for their future appointments, which was helpful for patient–provider communication, except for the challenge of orienting the camera.

GJ has experienced technical issues with VRI for not only D/HH patients, but also other LEP patients. She felt frustrated with VRI because it was difficult to communicate and make the patients feel comfortable, which resulted in emotional disconnection. In some instances, the iPad microphone did not work and caused a delay, since it was difficult to hear over the noisy background in the dental clinic.

Moreover, GJ has used in-person interpreters, which offered more effective patient–provider communication. However, they were rare due to the hospital's budget concerns. She also explained how difficult it is to communicate while wearing a mask. In this regard, she mentioned that her co-worker who was fluent in ASL did not have a translucent mask, but he used his hands and eyes to enable patient–provider communication. For example, he would fill in the information (when necessary) by using his hands or intermittently take off his mask to discuss everything first and then put the mask on during the treatment.

Finally, GJ suggested training to help healthcare providers understand patients' languages and the Deaf culture, to connect with their patients, and to provide small tips such as about removing a mask to show facial expressions, positioning the VRI equipment, and identifying appropriate times to use the device. GJ emphasized,

Sometimes, I have in-person interpreters and sometimes I have iPad video/audio interpreters for the English as a second language patients. I would definitely say that in-person is much better, but I think it is rarer because it is more expensive for institutions.

4.2.4 GO

GO is a 30-year-old female who has worked as a physical therapist for two years. She also teaches physical therapy students. She has experience in treating one deaf patient through VRI and caring for LEP patients through in-person interpreters.

When GO first saw the VRI unit, she thought that it was easy to use, i.e., she just had to log in and select the patient's language. Although she encountered poor connectivity, she had a good overall experience with the VRI. She mentioned that in-person interpreters would be useful for physical therapy because her patients are placed in different positions and constantly asked to move around. In this regard, it is not feasible to use VRI in such situations.

When GO used VRI, she prepared for the call ahead of time by explaining to the interpreter what positions the patients were going to be in before the treatments began. During the treatments, if the patients were lying face down, then she would ask them to hold their hand up if they felt pain. Thus, the patient–provider communication was arranged with the VRI interpreter beforehand:

I do not have a lot of experience, but I would be comfortable seeing more [deaf patients]…I think that it has improved over the time that I have been here. I also think that the majority of the patients feel comfortable using it [VRI]. So, I think that it works pretty well, as long as the connection is not poor.

4.2.5 MN

MN is a 38-year-old female who has worked as a nurse practitioner in emergency medicine for 15 years. She has treated D/HH patients who come to the emergency room at unexpected times and has frequently experienced situations where there is no interpreter available. In fact, she has never used an in-person interpreter but has used a patient's family member or friend for translation during emergency procedures. This was until the hospital introduced VRI several years ago.

In a recent interaction with VRI, MN saw a five-year-old deaf child with a cochlear implant and his mother with LEP. MN needed multiple interpreters to help communicate with both the boy and his mother. Accordingly, she used an English-Spanish onsite interpreter and an English-ASL VRI interpreter. Her experience was as follows:

The boy spoke English, or understood English and Spanish, but also utilized American Sign Language as his primary mode of communication. However, the mother primarily used Spanish. So, we had to use the video interpreter to help. The boy was a fairly adept, intelligent five-year-old who came in with ear pain. In this case, the video interpreter was extremely useful because we could talk to him directly, as opposed to me talking to a translator who translated to the mother, who then translated to the child.

Moreover, MN mentioned that VRI was used to treat adult D/HH patients for brief procedures, but it was difficult to move the VRI unit around when her patients moved between multiple rooms. She ended up using the written method to communicate with them. Thus, even though it is ideal to use an in-person interpreter, it is not feasible.

4.2.6   KS

KS is a 26-year-old male who has worked as an oral surgeon for two years. He has treated D/HH patients in different clinics. In his experience, the best mode of communication has been the type that the patient is the most comfortable using. In one instance, a patient completely refused to use a translator and wanted to communicate via note writing. He has also had some patients who preferred an in-person interpreter or VRI.

KS found that note writing can be an effective method because it eliminates the bias of the third-party interpreter. However, he has had particularly good experiences using in-person interpreters because it allows him to talk directly with the patient, without wondering if the VRI interpreter is capturing what he is saying.

KS has used VRI multiple times and has yet to like the approach. There have been obvious technical difficulties, and he feels like these take away from the dentist–patient interaction, trust, and relationship. In many instances, KS has had to maneuver the iPad to capture both himself and the patient in the field of view. This is somewhat difficult to do while performing a long procedure such as a root canal.

KS also emphasized that the benefit of using an in-person interpreter is that it allows for much more patient–provider interaction and leads to more treatment acceptance and a better treatment outcome. Whether it is a checkup or an urgent visit, an in-person interpreter always allows for the human trust connection. Moreover, KS stated that most patients do not really want to come in to see him and have work done, but if a trust relationship exists, then the chances of successful and compliant treatment are greater. KS concluded,

> Communication is probably one of the most important aspects of healthcare. So, having proper modes of communication for all languages is important.

4.2.7   TY

TY is a 27-year-old female who has worked as an obstetrics and gynecology nurse practitioner for 15 years. She has never used in-person interpreters but has employed a VRI computer mounted on the wall of a room. In some instances, she has used a patient's family member or friend as an interpreter. In this regard, she noticed that a family interpreter is not effective when they are unfamiliar with medical terminology. She was also unaware of the ethical and legal problems of using relatives as interpreters in medical settings. Since her clinic only has one VRI device, it can be time-consuming for other D/HH patients or LEP patients to wait for their turn to use it. She also shared the following:

> I know that one of my colleagues has and will write back and forth with the patients, especially when she is unable to obtain an interpreter. However, I do not know how effective this approach can be during treatment.

TY has also experienced communication barriers with her D/HH patients during gynecological exams. For example, one patient did not feel comfortable with the VRI interpreter appearing on the screen, so she had trouble communicating with her. TY prefers using a movable VRI device to obscure the patient's private parts during a gynecological exam. Thus, the appropriateness of the type of VRI, i.e., mounted or movable, depends on the type of clinical procedure.

4.2.8   WD

WD is a 50-year-old male who has worked as an orthopedic surgeon for 19 years. He has treated D/HH patients using both VRI and in-person interpreters. He once cared for a patient who read lips and communicated without signing. He also had another D/HH patient whose mother served as the interpreter. In other words, he accepts the patient's preference.

WD also explained that he sees no difference between D/HH patients and LEP patients. For both, it takes more time to establish and develop patient–provider communication. In his opinion, it is important that his patients understand their condition and what the treatment options are so that they can make a collaborative decision on the best course of treatment. He stated,

> You must remember to keep it simple and open and give the patient plenty of opportunities to ask questions. You also have to realize that it is going to take some extra time to communicate with them.

WD also expressed that VRI is economically viable. His private clinic struggles with its legal obligations, since it is forced to pay for interpreter services (as stipulated in the Americans with Disabilities Act). Moreover, the clinic loses money on LEP patients or D/HH patients because it does not receive reimbursements for the increased expenses of providing these services.

4.3 Conclusion

4.3.1 Comparison of Experiences with Video Remote Interpreting and In-Person Interpreting

Overall, EP, EK, GO, MN, TY, and WD had positive experiences with the use of VRI because it is convenient to access when an in-person interpreter is unavailable, whereas BE, EP, GJ, GO, KS, and TY had negative experiences because of VRI technology issues. MN and TY only had VRI at their respective clinics, and they often ended up using written communication methods or family interpreting when VRI was unavailable.

In addition, GO, EP, and KS had positive experiences with in-person interpreting services because they were able to achieve effective patient–provider communication and greater treatment outcomes. Conversely, MN found it difficult to obtain an in-person interpreter for emergency care.

4.3.2 Comparison of Interpreting Preferences for Critical and Non-critical Care

When discussing interpreting preferences for critical care, TY preferred using VRI because her clinic did not have staff interpreters, while EP and MN pointed out that it was unrealistic to expect to obtain an in-person interpreter for an emergency. In contrast, GJ, KS, and WD preferred using in-person interpreters because they were concerned about communication access during surgery.

As for non-critical care, GO and TY preferred VRI because their clinics already had it available. However, EP, KS, TY, and WD still preferred in-person interpreters because it offered better opportunities for successful and compliant treatment and effective communication for patients with cognitive disabilities.

4.3.3 Healthcare Professionals' Recommendations

Overall, BE, DO, GJ, GO, KS, and MN suggested that there is a need for improvement in VRI equipment and training, and more bilingual providers. GJ, GO, KS, and MN suggested upgrading VRI technology by improving connectivity, gaining more flexibility to move the device around, having a gooseneck attachment for selecting the correct height for users to see the screen better, having a larger screen for better visibility, and having brighter lighting for dental care.

BE suggested hiring more bilingual providers to achieve better patient–provider communication, while EP and GJ advocated for training students and providers to interact with D/HH patients using different interpreting modalities. They also suggested providing training for D/HH patients and their families about how to advocate for their rights.

Even though the healthcare professionals recognized that in-person interpreting provides better patient–provider communication than VRI, they eventually used VRI or written communication due to the hospital administration system, budget concerns, time constraints, and limited in-person interpreter availability.

Moreover, although the healthcare professionals were concerned with quality care, other factors such as cost and familiarity shaped their decisions about the use of VRI versus in-person interpreting. For the healthcare professionals, communication was not adversely impacted because they still communicated with the patients. However, they were less aware of how much (or little) the D/HH patients understood and interpreted the information. While most of the healthcare professionals lacked Deaf knowledge, they still recognized that the quality of patient–provider communication closely influenced treatment outcomes and healthcare experiences.

Appendix: Comparison Between Limited English Proficiency Patients and Deaf and Hard of Hearing Patients

Both limited English proficiency (LEP) and deaf and hard of hearing (D/HH) populations experience communication barriers due to a lack of qualified interpreters, providers' limited knowledge of cultural competency and their legal obligations, and limited literacy skills (Brooks et al., 2016; Chen et al., 2007; Harmer, 1999; Meador & Zazove, 2005). Meanwhile, healthcare providers often depend on ad hoc interpreters for LEP patients and D/HH patients, including the parents or children of LEP patients and D/HH patients (Harmer, 1999).

Even when interpreting services are available, LEP patients may turn them down due to time constraints or mistrust. Additionally, LEP patients may feel frustration and embarrassment at their limited language skills and attempt to express themselves in imperfect English in order to avoid depending on others' help. Sometimes, LEP patients may pretend that they understand the information (Brooks et al., 2016).

Meanwhile, D/HH patients experience similar frustration and pretend to understand the information given by providers. LEP and D/HH patients experience similar barriers to healthcare access, although LEP patients are better able to access healthcare communication with their family members in their native languages compared to D/HH patients with hearing family members (Harmer, 1999). This is because LEP patients have family members who are fluent in their native languages, compared to 90% of D/HH patients whose parents are hearing and often not fluent in sign languages. Hence, D/HH patients may have limited communication access at home (Mitchell & Karchmer, 2004).

Previous research examined the language skills of LEP and D/HH patients and found that both groups had significant difficulty understanding medical vocabulary. Moreover, D/HH patients expressed that their healthcare providers understood them less often than LEP patients. Yet, D/HH patients were less likely to re-explain themselves (McEwen & Anton-Culver, 1988).

According to the interviews with the eight healthcare professionals (BE, EP, GJ, GO, MN, KS, TY, and WD), there were similarities in patient–provider communication and financial concerns. Even though in-person interpreting is generally helpful for LEP patients and D/HH patients, there was no difference between the two groups in this regard because both experienced language challenges and required time for communication access. Meanwhile, the necessity of paying for in-person interpreting services had a negative impact on both populations (Yabe, 2019).

Finally, there were different challenges when working with LEP and D/HH patients. For example, for LEP patients, it was less challenging to use VRI because they could hear when they would lie down or move round. However, for D/HH patients, it was more challenging to use VRI because they were unable to see the interpreter in such instances. Therefore, the decision to use different interpreting modalities is driven by logistics and the type of language accommodations that each of these populations requires (Yabe, 2019).

References

Brooks, K., Stifani, B., Batlle, H. R., Nunez, M. A., Erlich, M., & Diaz, J. (2016). Patient perspectives on the need for and barriers to professional medical interpretation. *Rhode Island Medical Journal, 4*(99), 30–33. https://www.rimed.org/rimedicaljournal/2016/01/2016-01-30-cont-brooks.pdf

Chen, A. H., Youdelman, M. K., & Brooks, J. (2007). The legal framework for language access in healthcare settings: Title VI and beyond. *Journal of General Internal Medicine, 22*(2), 362–367. https://doi.org/10.1007/s11606-007-0366-2

Harmer, L. M. (1999). Health care delivery and deaf people: Practice, problems, and recommendations for change. *Journal of Deaf Studies and Deaf Education, 4*(2), 73–110. https://doi.org/10.1093/deafed/4.2.73

McEwen, E., & Anton-Culver, H. (1988). The medical communication of deaf patients. *Journal of Family Practice, 26*(3), 289–291.

Meador, H. E., & Zazove, P. (2005). Health care interactions with deaf culture. *Journal of the American Board of Family Medicine, 18*(3), 218–222. https://doi.org/10.3122/jabfm.18.3.218

Mitchell, R. E., & Karchmer, M. A. (2004). Chasing the mythical ten percent: Parental hearing status of deaf and hard of hearing students in the United States. *Sign Language Studies, 4*(2), 138–163. https://doi.org/10.1353/sls.2004.000510.1353/sls.2004.0005

Yabe, M. (2019). *Healthcare providers' and deaf patients' perspectives on video remote interpreting: A mixed methods study* [Doctoral dissertation, University of Illinois Chicago]. University Library. http://hdl.handle.net/10027/23667

Chapter 5

Conclusion and Implications

> After my car accident, I received my first physical therapy treatment. For communication access, my first treatmnt relied on writing. It took nearly two hours for intake.
>
> My second treatment relied on VRI. My physical therapist logged in to call a VRI interpreter, and he explained to me what to do during the treatment. Then, he turned the VRI device off, and we started the treatment without VRI. At the end of the session, he called them again and obtained a different VRI interpreter. It was better than writing since my treatment was completed in an hour. We continued using VRI for several weeks. But I decided to ask my physical therapist to try using an in-person interpreter.
>
> My sixth treatment relied on an in-person interpreter. At the end of the session, my physical therapist told me,
>
> "Thank you for suggesting that I request an in-person interpreter. I realized how much an in-person interpreter is the BEST at communication, compared to VRI!"

5.1 Introduction

The excerpt above is my personal reflection as a deaf patient. Overall, I have used various communication methods, including writing, VRI, and in-person interpreting during physical therapy. After trying these different methods, my physical therapist and I agreed to use an in-person interpreter because it yielded the best patient–provider communication.

In this final chapter, I offer recommendations and justifications for hospital administrators, VRI companies, healthcare professionals, and medical educators and their students. I hope that readers will find the insights and guidance beneficial for providing excellent care.

M. Yabe, *Deaf Rhetoric*, SpringerBriefs in Public Health,
https://doi.org/10.1007/978-3-030-96245-6_5

5.2   Concluding Remarks

5.2.1   Hospital Administrators

Overall, I underscore my main research finding that economics and the ignorance of the "hearing society" toward the Deaf community, Deaf people, and Deaf culture have pushed hospital administrators toward a "common sense" conclusion that VRI is the best overall option. However, this is a faulty interpretation. My research reveals that VRI has limitations to ensuring patient–provider communication due to technology issues, limited placement and mobility, and a lack of human trust relationship, compared to in-person interpreting (Yabe, 2019).

Accordingly, hospital administrators should not rely soley on VRI for clinical procedures, but they should also allocate funding for in-person interpreting for critical care encounters such as emergency medicine, surgery, cognitive speech therapy, and cancer treatment.

In addition, my research identifies not only the perspectives of D/HH patients but also those of healthcare professionals on VRI versus in-person interpreting. Hospital administrators and VRI companies in the USA must adhere to their legal obligations and provide training for not only healthcare providers, staff, and VRI interpreters, but also for D/HH patients and their families to increase patient self-advocacy (Yabe, 2019).

Researching communication access in healthcare environments and spotlighting VRI and in-person interpreting also clarifies that more research is necessary. For instance, several questions are raised: (a) Are VRI interpreters more likely to break the code of ethics, and are they less prepared than in-person interpreters? (b) What are the perspectives of hard of hearing patients who are non-signers on VRI and in-person interpreting? and (c) What are the perspectives of non-deaf LEP patients on VRI and in-person interpreting? Future studies should answer these questions in addition to determining the cost-effectiveness of VRI and in-person interpreting.

Most importantly, hospital administrators must reframe their perspective on how to improve the quality of healthcare services that lead to better treatment outcomes and patient–provider communication. My research also points out that good practices in healthcare research and many other fields underscore that access and design are processes, not checklists. Engaging with the people most impacted (in this case, D/HH patients) and seeking their input on a regular basis can enable healthcare professionals to address barriers, improve trust, and cultivate better outcomes.

5.2.2   Video Remote Interpreting Companies

As my research consistently reveals, VRI companies' policies/practices and the equipment used for VRI warrant greater attention. In this regard, VRI companies must work closely with hospital administrators to improve the quality of VRI equipment as well as undertake initiatives to provide medical training for VRI inter-preters. Future studies are also necessary to confirm how many VRI interpreters are medically trained. In my literature review, one article reports higher levels of burn-out among video relay services interpreters, which can increase the risk of transla-tion errors (Bower, 2015). However, I found no other articles on the same topic related to VRI interpreters. Therefore, VRI companies and VRI interpreters must adopt a new perspective on how to improve the quality of VRI services. This can lead to improvements in patient–provider communication and better treatment results.

5.2.3   Healthcare Professionals

Healthcare professionals must be aware of how ecological factors (i.e., physical-material, spatial, psychological, social, and temporal dimensions) can influence patient–provider communication, treatment outcomes, and healthcare experiences in order to determine the best option for their patients and clinics. Some healthcare professionals believe that VRI services can save money in comparison to in-person interpreting services.

Interestingly, in my research, there was a conflict related to budget concerns between healthcare professionals and D/HH patients. Specifically, the healthcare professionals valued VRI because it seemed economical, whereas the D/HH patients saw it as wasteful because its quality was lower than in-person interpreting. In other words, it was about money for the healthcare professionals and about access for the D/HH patients. In this regard, financial factors that cloud the larger ethical and pro-fessional goals of quality care must be addressed.

These concerns are closely linked with the political economy of the healthcare system in the USA, i.e., the imperative for cost control, quick services, efficiency under managed care, and a for-profit health system. This system, which at one point was supposed to provide universal health care, was changed to an inequality-based healthcare system due to the enforcement of corporate power and economic crises. As a result, the healthcare system has become a medical marketplace where private care providers can engage in unrestricted commerce with patients as consumers (Gaffney, 2015).

In this situation, expenses depend on the costs demanded by VRI companies and specific situations. Additionally, if VRI fails due to poor connectivity, patients must reschedule another meeting and request an in-person interpreter, which can result in a loss of the patients' time and their healthcare insurance reimbursement. Meanwhile, the hospital administration would waste time and money paying for VRI services at the initial appointment and still make additional payments for in-person interpreting at the next appointment. Hence, healthcare professionals and administrators would benefit from reframing the idea of using VRI into a new per-spective about how better patient–provider communication can lead to better treat-ment outcomes.

5.2.4 Medical Educators and Students

Overall, the evidence points to training. My research and other related studies collectively show that training would benefit medical schools because effective patient–provider communication can result in improved treatment outcomes, human trust relationships, and healthcare experiences. Medical schools must also add Deaf Studies and Disability Studies curricula to educate future healthcare professionals to communicate with patients with disabilities and D/HH patients, train them in appropriately using an in-person interpreter and VRI interpreter, and increase their awareness of Deaf culture.

In fact, when I first presented a pilot Disability Studies workshop for the College of Medicine at the University of Illinois, Chicago, a medical student approached me and expressed interest in supporting the curriculum. One year later, the medical student helped lead the introduction of a Disability Studies curriculum and invited me as a guest speaker. In the following year, incoming medical students with disabilities joined and led the Disability Studies curriculum. It is important to note that if medical schools do not have these resources, then healthcare professional students can advocate for themselves and establish a disability workshop for students as well as a support group for healthcare professional students with disabilities.

5.3 Implications

Overall, this book emphasizes the value of process and the need to engage with D/HH communities, organizations, and institutions. This is specifically aimed at medical educators, healthcare practitioners, hospital administrators, healthcare professional students, and medical interpreters. Most importantly, healthcare communities must learn how to collaborate with D/HH patients and choose the best practices for improving patient–provider communication in any situation.

References

Bower, K. (2015). Stress and burnout in video relay services (VRS) interpreting. *Journal of Interpreting, 24*(1), 1–16. https://digitalcommons.unf.edu/joi/vol24/iss1/2/

Gaffney, A. W. (2015). The neoliberal turn in American health care. *International Journal of Health Services, 45*(1), 33–52. https://doi.org/10.2190/hs.45.1.d

Yabe, M. (2019). *Healthcare providers' and deaf patients' perspectives on video remote interpreting: A mixed methods study* [Doctoral dissertation, University of Illinois Chicago]. University Library. http://hdl.handle.net/10027/23667

Index

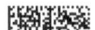